Anatomical Principles of Endoscopic Sinus Surgery: A Step by Step Approach

With warm regards,

R Bradoo
21/9/12

System requirement:
- **Windows XP or above**
- **Power DVD player (Software)**
- **Windows media player 11.0 version or above (Software)**

Accompanying CD ROM is playable only in Computer and not in CD player.

Kindly wait for few seconds for CD ROM to autorun. If it does not autorun then please do the following:
- Click on my computer
- Click the **CD/DVD drive** and after opening the drive, kindly double click the file **Jaypee**

Index for VCD (Endoscopic Anatomy)

Anatomical Principles of Endoscopic Sinus Surgery: A Step by Step Approach

Renuka Bradoo

MS DORL

Professor and Head
Department of ENT
and
Head and Neck Surgery
Lokmanya Tilak Municipal Medical College
and General Hospital
Sion, Mumbai

FORWORD
MV Kirtane

JAYPEE BROTHERSS MEDICAL PUBLISHERS (P) LTD

New Delhi • Panama City • London

Jaypee Brothers Medical Publishers (P) Ltd

Headquarter

Jaypee Brothers Medical Publishers (P) Ltd
4838/24, Ansari Road, Daryaganj
New Delhi 110 002, India
Phone: +91-11-43574357
Fax: +91-11-43574314
Email: jaypee@jaypeebrothers.com

Overseas Offices

JP Medical Ltd
83 Victoria Street, London
SW1H 0HW (UK)
Phone: +44-2031708910
Fax: +02-03-0086180
Email: info@jpmedpub.com

Jaypee-Highlights Medical Publishers Inc
City of Knowledge, Bld. 237, Clayton
Panama City, Panama
Phone: 507-301-0496
Fax: +50-73-010499
Email: cservice@jphmedical.com

Website: www.jaypeebrothers.com
Website: www.jaypeedigital.com

Inquiries for bulk sales may be solicited at: jaypee@jaypeebrothers.com

This book has been published in good faith that the contents provided by the contributors contained herein are original, and is intended for educational purposes only. While every effort is made to ensure accuracy of information, the publisher and the editor specifically disclaim any damage, liability, or loss incurred, directly or indirectly, from the use or application of any of the contents of this work. If not specifically stated, all figures and tables are courtesy of the editor. Where appropriate, the readers should consult with a specialist or contact the manufacturer of the drug or device.

Anatomical Principles of Endoscopic Sinus Surgery: A Step by Step Approach

First Edition: 2005
Reprint: **2012**

ISBN 81-8061-346-1

Printed at Ajanta Offset & Packgings Ltd., New Delhi

Dedicated
to

Anil
For being both my anchor and the wind in my sails

Anjali and Anant Savant
My parents
For translating my dreams into reality

Mohini and Mohanlal Bradoo
My in-laws
For their unstinting support always

And
Rishi and Hriday
Who make it all worthwhile

Foreword

Endoscopic Sinus Surgery (ESS) has progressed immensely in the last 2 decades. The interest in the subject and the desire to acquire proficiency in the surgical technique has led to enthusiastic attendance at numerous 'workshops' being conducted in India and abroad. The introduction of motorized instruments, laser, image guided surgery etc., and the evolving concepts of the 'right way' to do the surgery are steps to making this procedure as 'functional' as possible. The basic need of the aspiring surgeon however, is still an accurate knowledge of the anatomy of the region, a 3 dimensional concept, which will allow him to approach and clear disease from the narrow recesses of the nose and the paranasal sinuses and restore function to near normal.

Dr Renuka Bradoo, who is currently the Professor and Head, Department of ENT and Head and Neck Surgery at the Lokmanya Tilak Municipal Medical College and General Hospital, Mumbai, has been an outstanding teacher, a skilled surgeon and a brilliant speaker as evidenced by the numerous lectures and workshops she has conducted in ESS.

She has been interested in the subject for many years. This book authored by her exemplifies her methodical approach and the tremendous efforts she has put into make it as complete as possible. The book has been well planned and carries several colored illustrations of very high quality. The text in the various chapters is excellent in its clarity of presentation. I am confident that this book will be of immense value to all aspiring and established sinus surgeons.

Dr MV Kirtane
Mumbai

Preface

This book was not planned to be written. It grew out of my experience and took on an identity of its own. Over the last few years, I have been guest faculty at various endoscopic sinus surgery workshops throughout the country besides conducting workshops at my own institution. One of the lectures I am often asked to take is the one on the anatomy of lateral nasal wall. Almost invariably, after the lecture various colleagues would approach me to know where they could access the material I had just discussed, on a regular basis. It was then, that I realized the need for a book dedicated exclusively to anatomy of the nose and paranasal sinuses as viewed by an endoscopic surgeon. It also went hand in hand with my absolute belief that to be a safe but effective endoscopic sinus surgeon one needs to have a very strong foundation of anatomy. In fact, the entire skull should be mapped in 3-dimensional form in the surgeon's brain. It is with this in mind that I have written a separate chapter on osteology.

Two chapters which complement each other include the anatomy of the Lateral Nasal Wall as seen in sagittal section and the Endoscopic Anatomy as seen by the surgeon in a live patient. These are illustrated in a stepwise manner. The chapter on Endoscopic Anatomy is accompanied by a CD-ROM.

Another prerequisite of a clinically sound surgeon is that he should be able to read the fine nuances of a CT scan of the paranasal sinuses. Anyone can say whether the sinuses are diseased or normal. What is required is to have a detailed knowledge of both normal findings and anatomical variations seen on the CT scan so that it can be used as a compass or road map during surgery. I have therefore included two chapters, one on reading the normal CT scan and a separate one on deviations from the normal.

The chapter on surgical anatomy is more of a summary of different facts that we already know or should know, put together in one comprehensive capsule.

The first chapter, very suitably, deals with embryology of the nose and paranasal sinuses because '….he sees things best who sees them from the beginning'. It answers in many cases- the reason why?

I have tried to illustrate the book extensively using cadaveric dissection specimens with explanatory line diagrams alongside. There are also endoscopic pictures, CT scans and schematic diagrams.

I hope this book proves to be useful to you and that you enjoy reading it as much as I have enjoyed writing it.

Renuka Bradoo

Acknowledgements

The book has my name on its cover, but I owe this effort to many people who have touched my life in so many ways.

I would like to thank all my patients who have been my first and foremost teachers. Dr Gadre, Dr Bhargava and Dr Morwani, my teachers in the formal sense, opened up the vistas of ENT for me. I have learnt a great deal from Dr Kirtane, whom I think of as a guru. Dr Dale Rice first sparked off my interest in endoscopic sinus surgery when I watched him operate on his visit to India. I never cease to be amazed by the poetry of Dr Sethi's surgery. Watching him has helped me to fine tune many of my surgical techniques.

I have been fortunate in having an excellent faculty in my department—Dr Nerurkar, Dr Joshi and Dr Kalel. They have held the fort whenever I have been away and made valuable suggestions. I also take this opportunity to thank my residents and Dr Sujata Muranjan for the numerous times that they have burnt the midnight oil with me. Dr Mishra helped me research the first chapter of Embryology. My very special thanks to Dr Jayesh Shah, my student and now my colleague without whose hard work and persistence this book would have remained just a dream and never have seen the light of the day.

There are a myriad of technical inputs which go into making a book like this one. I would like to thank M/s Chimco Biomedical and Infometry for helping me to shoot the endoscopic images, Mr Khan and Mr Chandrakant Desai for photographing the cadaveric images and Mr Krishna Patil and Ganesh for the artwork. Dr PP Rao helped me with digitizing the images. Mrs Lakshmi Nakhawa was invaluable as always for her secretarial help and her down to earth common sense. The "other" Lakshmi, Ms Lakshmi Perla typed the manuscript many times over.

I owe my thanks to various Heads of Departments—Dr Athaviya, Head, Department of Anatomy and Dr Pathak, Head, Department of Forensic Medicine for providing me cadavers on which I could conduct my dissections and research, Dr Merchant and Dr Joshi of the Department of Radiology for letting me choose CT scans from their archives. I would also like to thank, Dr ME Yeolekar, Dean, Lokmanya Tilak Municipal Medical College and General Hospital.

On a personal note, my family and friends have always been a tremendous support system cushioning me in my setbacks and rejoicing in my triumphs.

Contents

Abbreviations

A	Atrium
AEA	Anterior ethmoid artery
AEC	Anterior ethmoid cell
Ag	Agger nasi
AO	Accessory ostium
B	Bulla ethmoidalis
CG	Crista galli
EO	Eustachian tube opening
FS	Frontal sinus
FI	Frontal infundibulum
FO	Frontal ostium
FR	Frontal recess
GL	Ground lamella
HSI	Hiatus semilunaris inferioris
HSS	Hiatus semilunaris superioris
I	Infundibulum
ICA	Internal carotid artery
IT	Inferior turbinate
LP	Lamina papyracea
MO	Maxillary ostium
MR	Medial rectus
MS	Maxillary sinus
MT	Maxillary turbinate
NLD	Nasolacrimal duct
ON	Optic nerve
PEA	Posterior ethmoid artery
PEC	Posterior ethmoid cell
Pit	Pituitary
PPF	Pterygopalatine fossa
S	Septum
SER	Sphenoethmoidal recess
SL	Sinus lateralis
SO	Sphenoid ostium
SS	Sphenoid sinus
ST	Superior turbinate
U	Uncinate process
V	Vestibule

Embryology

*"He who sees things grow from the beginning,
will have the finest view of them"*
—Aristotle (384-322 BC)

1

Embryology

The development of the nose and paranasal sinuses needs to be studied in conjunction with the development of the face, in order to have a complete understanding of the subject. Facial development takes place mainly between the 4th and 8th weeks of intrauterine life, during which time a mass of undifferentiated swellings at the head end of the fetus undergo growth and remodelling to form a distinctly recognizable human profile. The face develops from five facial swellings that surround the stomodeum or primitive mouth by the end of the 4th week. The swellings consist of a central unpaired process called the frontonasal process, a pair of maxillary and a pair of mandibular processes. The maxillary and mandibular processes are both sub-divisions of the first pharyngeal arch. The frontonasal process is the downward proliferation of the ectoderm over the forebrain (Fig. 1.1).

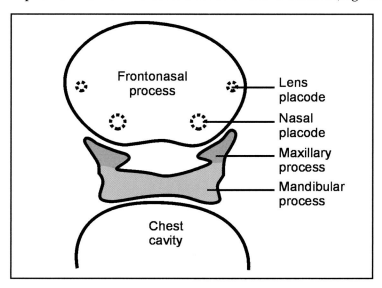

Fig. 1.1: The 5-week embryo—formation of facial processes

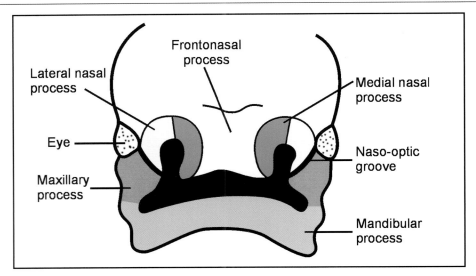

Fig. 1.2: The 6-week embryo

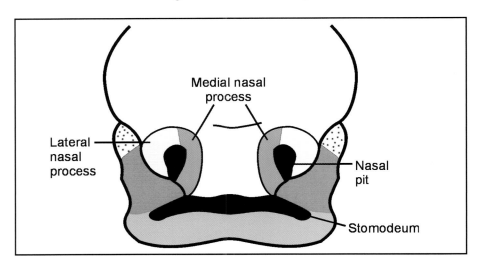

Fig. 1.3: The 7-week embryo—medial migration of maxillary process

During the 5th week, a pair of ectodermal thickenings appear on the frontonasal process. These are called the nasal placodes. In the 6th week, the ectoderm in the center of each nasal placode invaginates to form an oval nasal pit. The raised rims of these nasal pits form the lateral and medial nasal processes (Fig. 1.2). During the 6th and 7th weeks, the maxillary processes on either side increase in size and grow medially. This medial migration of the maxillary processes causes the medial nasal processes to move towards each other. As the maxillary processes grow medially, they fuse first with the lateral nasal process and then with the medial nasal process. This separates the nasal pits from the stomodeum (Fig. 1.3).

The medial nasal processes fuse with each other to form the intermaxillary process. The central tissues of the intermaxillary process get pushed upwards to form the nasal prominence characteristic of human beings. The inter-maxillary process forms the central bridge of the nose and the central portion

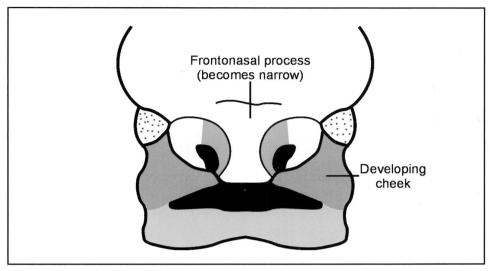

Fig. 1.4: Medial nasal processes fuse to form intermaxillary process.
Maxillary and mandibular process fuse to form cheek

of the upper lip called the philtrum (Fig. 1.4). At the end of the 6th week, the nasal pits deepen and coalesce to form a single cavity behind the intermaxillary process. This cavity is initially separated from the stomodeum lying below it by a thin membrane called the oronasal membrane. This membrane ruptures during the 7th week to form the primitive choana, which is the opening of the primitive nasal cavity into the stomodeum or developing mouth (Figs 1.5A and B).

The intermaxillary process grows backward to form the nasal septum. The lateral nasal processes enlarge to form the nasal alae. They also grow backwards to form the lateral nasal wall. This developing lateral nasal wall

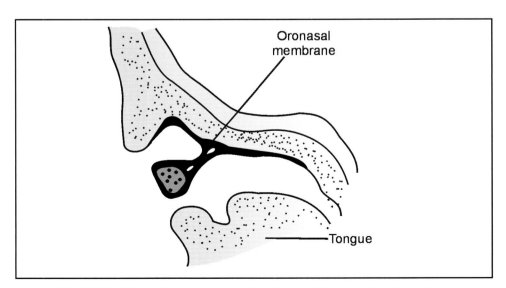

Fig. 1.5A: A 6-week embryo—showing the primitive nasal cavity which is separated from the oral cavity by the oronasal membrane

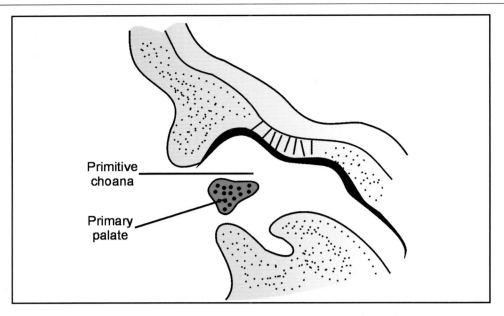

Fig. 1.5B: A 7-week embryo—breakdown of oronasal membrane

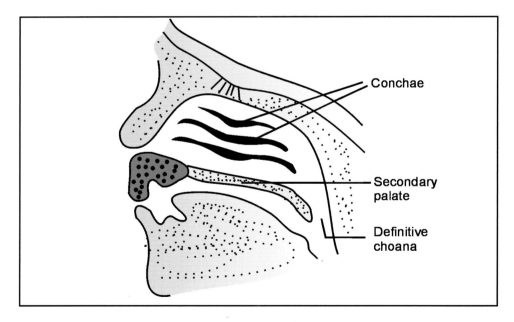

Fig. 1.6: A 9-week embryo—formation of secondary
palate and definitive choana

shows multiple anteroposterior elevations, which are finally reduced to three or occasionally four in number. These are the turbinates, which overhang corresponding meatii (Fig. 1.6).

The maxillary processes fuse with the lateral nasal processes. The junction of their fusion is marked by a groove called the nasolacrimal or naso-optic groove. By the 7th week, this groove invaginates into the underlying mesenchyme to form the nasolacrimal duct. The canalization of nasolacrimal duct continues throughout pregnancy and may not be complete till after birth.

The floor of the nasal cavity, which is the hard palate, is formed during the 8th and 9th week. The medial surfaces of the maxillary processes form thin medial extensions called palatine shelves. These shelves first grow downwards on either side of the developing tongue; but by the end of the 9th week, they rotate upwards into a horizontal position. They then fuse with each other in the midline and with the primary palate anteriorly to form the secondary palate. The secondary palate also fuses with the lower border of the developing nasal septum. The nasal cavity is thus divided into two nasal passages, which open into the pharynx behind the secondary palate through openings called the definitive choanae (Figs 1.7A to C). The mandibular processes grow medially and fuse in the midline to form the lower lip and jaw.

On day 24, the buccopharyngeal membrane in the depths of the stomodeum ruptures to form a broad, slit-like embryonic mouth. The mouth is reduced to its final width during the second month as fusion of the lateral portion of the maxillary and mandibular processes create the cheeks.

At birth, the volume of the cranial vault is seven times the volume of the facial skeleton. This ratio steadily decreases during infancy and childhood. This is mainly as a result of the growth of four pairs of paranasal sinuses and the development of the teeth.

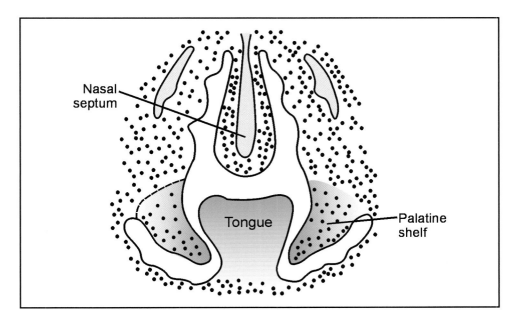

Fig. 1.7A: The 8-week embryo—formation of palatine shelves

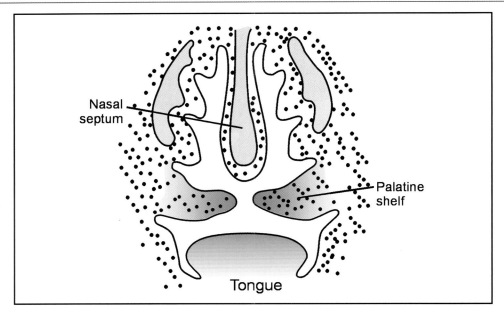

Fig. 1.7B: The 9-week embryo—rotation of palatine shelves

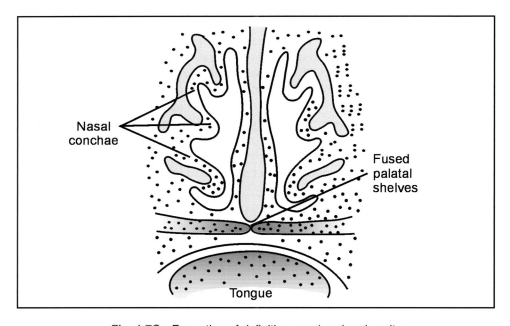

Fig. 1.7C: Formation of definitive nasal and oral cavity

Table 1.1: Structures contributing to formation of the face (Fig. 1.8)

Processes	Structures formed
Frontonasal	Forehead, bridge of nose, medial and lateral nasal prominences
Maxillary	Cheeks, lateral portion of upper lip
Medial nasal	Philtrum of upper lip, crest and tip of nose, septum
Lateral nasal	Alae of nose, lateral nasal wall
Mandibular	Lower lip and jaw

Fig. 1.8

The sinuses develop from invaginations of the nasal cavity that extend into the surrounding bones. The maxillary and ethmoid sinuses develop *in utero* during the 3rd and 5th fetal months respectively. The maxillary sinus is in the form of an elongated sac in the neonate. With the eruption of the deciduous teeth, it enlarges to become three times longer anteroposteriorly and five times greater in height and width. Thus, the floor of the maxillary sinus which is above the floor of the nasal cavity at birth, lies below it in adults. The ethmoid sinuses are small before the age of two years, then grow rapidly till 6 to 8 years but do not complete their growth until puberty.

Around the second year of life, the most anterior ethmoid cells grow into the frontal bone to form the frontal sinuses. The frontal sinuses are visible on X-rays by the seventh year of life. Between the second and fifth years, the most posterior ethmoid cells grow into the sphenoid bone to form the sphenoid sinus. The frontal sinuses do not start developing until the second postnatal year. Sphenoid sinuses do not usually develop until fifth year of life.

Growth of the paranasal sinuses not only changes the shape and the size of the face in childhood but also adds resonance to the voice in adolescence.

Osteology

"Don't loose the wood for the trees,
..... get the whole picture first!"

2 Osteology

There are two ways to study any concept:
The *swiss cheese* technique in which one picks out the important salient features first and gradually gets the idea of the whole concept. The second is the *building block* technique where one breaks down the whole concept into its component parts, studies each part separately and then puts it together again to form the whole picture. We will use this building block technique to study the complex anatomy of the lateral nasal wall.

The cadaveric head when cut in the immediate para-saggital plane reveals the lateral nasal wall. On first impression, this area appears as a series of elevations and depressions. The lateral nasal wall extends from the nasal vestibule to the posterior choana, which is formed by the medial surface of the medial pterygoid plate. The nasopharynx extends beyond the posterior choana up to the pre-vertebral muscles. What strikes us immediately is that the nasal airway extends up to approximately 50 percent of the distance of the entire sagittal section of the head (Fig. 2.1).

The nasal mucosa is stripped off the underlying bones (Figs 2.2A and B). We see that the lateral nasal wall is formed by eight separate bones, each of which have processes that articulate intricately with each other (Fig. 2.3). There are four large bones; the maxilla, the frontal, the ethmoid and the sphenoid, and four small bones; the inferior turbinate, the lacrimal, the palatine and the nasal bones. Of these, the frontal, ethmoid and sphenoid are single unpaired bones in the midline of the skull. The others are paired bones. Hence, although there are two sphenoid, two frontal and two ethmoid sinuses, there is only a single sphenoid, frontal and ethmoid bone. We will now disarticulate all the bones and study the relevant anatomy of each bone. Having done that we will re-articulate them to study the lateral nasal wall as a whole.

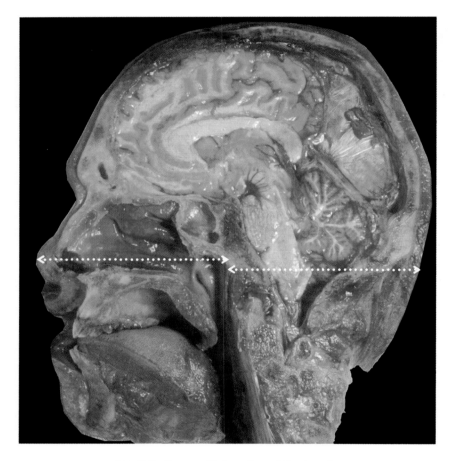

Fig. 2.1: Parasagittal section of the head

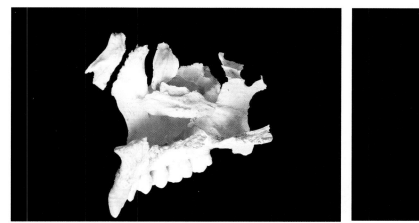
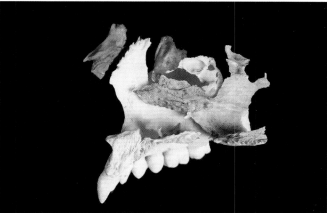

Figs 2.2A and B: Articulated bones that form part of the lateral nasal wall

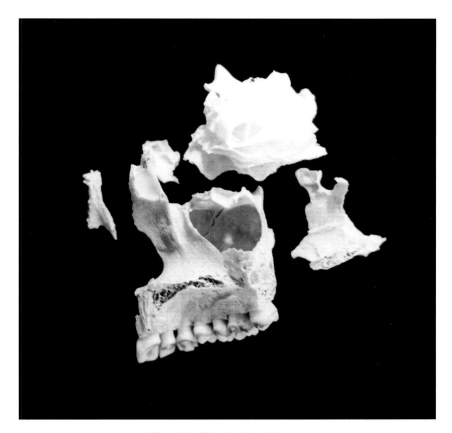

Fig. 2.3: Disarticulated bones

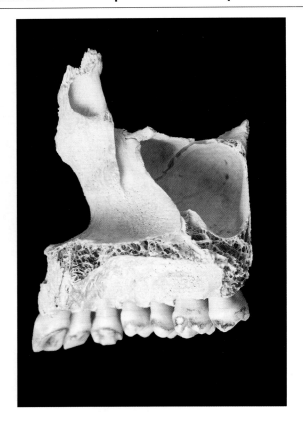

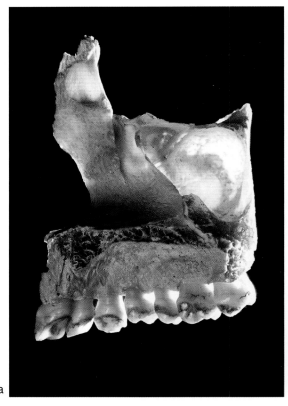

Figs 2.4A and B: Maxilla

The Maxilla (Figs 2.4A and B)

The maxilla forms the base or the framework on which the lateral nasal wall is built and so we will study it first. The lateral nasal wall is formed by the

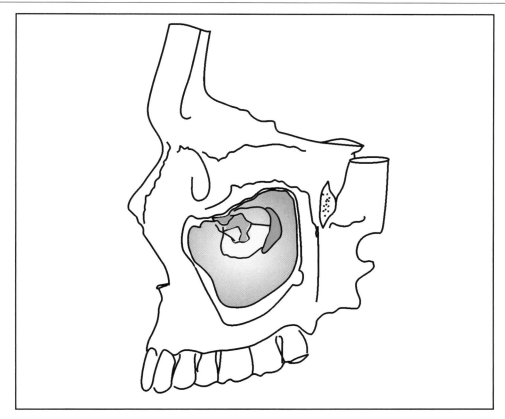

Fig. 2.5: Red—descending process of the lacrimal bone. Green—uncinate process. Yellow—maxillary process of the inferior turbinate. Blue—perpendicular plate of the palatine bone

medial surface of the maxilla. What is most obvious is a large opening into the maxillary sinus. We know that in the live patient the maxillary sinus opening is small and not easily seen. This is because the large opening in the maxillary bone is closed off by processes of different bones, which narrow the opening. These processes are:

- *The descending process* of the lacrimal bone anteriorly
- *The uncinate process* of the ethmoid bone anteroinferiorly
- *The maxillary process* of the inferior turbinate inferiorly
- *The perpendicular plate* of the palatine bone posteriorly (Fig. 2.5).

Certain areas are covered by only a double layer of mucosa of the nasal cavity and the maxillary sinus. These are the anterior and posterior fontanelles. Occasionally, these double layers of the mucosa may be dehiscent to produce accessory ostia. The normal maxillary ostium is hidden deep behind the intermediate portion of the uncinate process.

Anterior to the maxillary hiatus, the maxillary bone is drawn into a process, which extends superiorly. Since the upper border of this process articulates with the frontal bone and the anterior border articulates with the nasal bone, this process is called the frontonasal process of the maxilla. The medial surface of this process shows two crests. The upper one is the ethmoidal crest. The most anterior part of the middle turbinate is attached to this ethmoidal crest. The agger nasi cells also overlie this crest anterior to the attachment of the middle turbinate. Pneumatization of this part of the frontonasal process along with the adjacent lacrimal bone contributes to the formation of the agger nasi cells. The lower crest is called the conchal crest and gives attachment to the inferior turbinate. The smooth area below the conchal crest forms part of the inferior meatus.

Immediately behind the frontonasal process is a groove. This groove is closed by the lacrimal bone and the lacrimal process of the inferior turbinate to form a canal for the nasolacrimal duct. The frontonasal process is a thick bone, whilst the lacrimal bone is quite thin. Therefore, it is interesting to know that although the lateral wall of the nasolacrimal duct is formed by thick bone, its medial wall is formed by fairly thin bone, which can be easily damaged.

Posterior to the hiatus at the junction of the medial and the posterior wall of the maxilla is a roughened area called the maxillary tuberosity. This area has an oblique groove which when completed by the perpendicular plate of the palatine bone forms the canal for the greater palatine vessels and nerve.

The endoscopic surgeon must also understand the anatomy of the roof of the maxillary sinus and its posterior wall. The roof is formed by the orbital surface of the maxilla and is marked by the infraorbital canal, which may sometimes be dehiscent to expose its contents, namely, the infraorbital vessels and nerve. The posterolateral wall of the maxillary sinus is smooth and featureless and comprises of fairly thin bone. It separates the maxillary sinus from the pterygopalatine fossa medially and the infratemporal fossa laterally.

The Frontal Bone (Figs 2.6A and B)

The contribution of the frontal bone to the lateral nasal wall is best understood by looking at its basal view. In the centre of the bone is a hiatus, which is

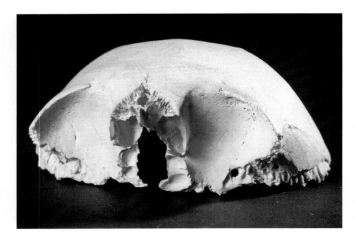

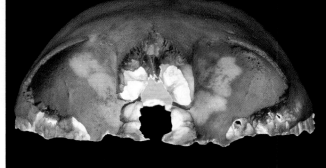

Figs 2.6A and B: Frontal bone

filled, in the living person by the cribriform plate of the ethmoid. On either side of this hiatus are a variable number of air cells. These are the anterior and posterior ethmoid air cells. The roof of these air cells is the skull base or the ethmoid fovea. Thus, the ethmoid fovea is at a higher level than the cribriform plate. The lateral border of these air cells articulates with the lamina papyracea of the ethmoid bone. It is at the junction of these suture lines between the lamina and the frontal bone that there exist the anterior and posterior ethmoidal foramina transmitting their respective arteries. Lateral to the lamina papyracea is the orbit. Anteriorly and in the midline, the frontal bone is elongated to form the nasal spine. This spine articulates with the nasal bones, which help in forming the anteriormost portion of the lateral nasal wall.

The Ethmoid Bone (Figs 2.7A and B)

The ethmoid bone is a single delicate bone consisting of numerous air cells—the ethmoidal sinuses. It consists of a horizontal plate, i.e. the cribriform plate and a vertical plate in the midline, i.e. the perpendicular plate. The perpendicular plate forms the posterior part of the septum.

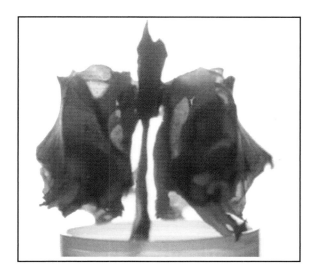

Fig. 2.7A: Ethmoid bone (coronal view)

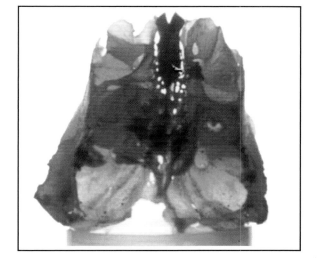

Fig. 2.7B: Ethmoid bone (axial view)

The cribriform plate fits into the notch in the frontal bone and separates the nose from the anterior cranial fossa, more specifically, the gyrus rectus and the olfactory bulb. It is perforated by many foramina, which transmit the olfactory nerves as well as the anterior and posterior ethmoidal arteries. On the upper surface of the cribriform plate in the midline is a projection, which is called the crista galli. The crista galli is occasionally pneumatized (Fig. 2.8). On closer examination, the cribriform plate shows a horizontal medial lamella and an oblique or vertical lateral lamella. This lateral lamella articulates with the frontal bone. Thus, the skull base in this region—the ethmoid fovea—is formed medially by the lateral lamella of the cribriform plate, which is very thin bone and laterally by the frontal bone, which in contrast is a thicker bone. The frontal

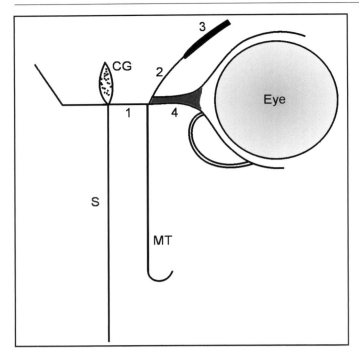

Fig. 2.8: The cribriform plate and ethmoid fovea: (1) Horizontal lamella, (2) Lateral lamella, (3) Orbital plate of frontal bone, (4) Anterior ethmoidal artery

bone forming the ethmoid fovea is 0.5 mm in thickness while the lateral lamella of the cribriform plate is 0.2 mm. The region where the anterior ethmoidal artery pierces the dura medially is the thinnest area in the base skull and is only 0.05 mm in thickness. The length of the lateral lamella and the depth of the olfactory fossa are classified by Keros into 3 types:

- Type I   —   1-3 mm
- Type II   —   4-7 mm
- Type III   —   8-17 mm

Lateral to the perpendicular plate on either side, are two masses of air cells—the ethmoidal sinuses (Fig. 2.9). They are bounded medially by the middle

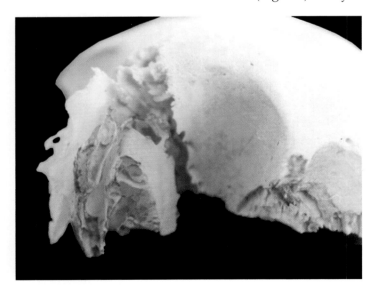

Fig. 2.9: The basal view of the articulated frontal and ethmoid bones: (1) perpendicular plate (white), (2) middle turbinate (blue), (3) uncinate process (green), (4) ethmoid air cells (yellow) and lamina papyracea

and superior turbinate and laterally by the paper-thin lamina papyracea, which separates the ethmoid from the orbit. Occasionally, there may be a supreme turbinate above the superior turbinate. It is important to know that although the inferior turbinate is a separate bone, the middle and superior turbinates are parts of the ethmoid bone. The middle turbinate overhangs a space called the middle meatus. Similarly, the space under the superior turbinate is the superior meatus.

The middle turbinate is a thin sheet of bone, which curves in different planes very similar to a dried leaf. Its most anterior attachment is in the sagittal plane to the frontonasal process of the maxilla and cribriform plate. It then turns laterally to be attached in the coronal plane to the lamina papyracea. This attachment is called the basal or ground lamella. Its most posterior attachment is in the horizontal plane along the lamina papyracea and the perpendicular plate of the palatine bone up to the roof of the posterior choana.

A gently curved bony process lies almost free within the middle meatus partially covering the maxillary sinus opening. This is the uncinate process. It articulates anteriorly with the lacrimal bone and at its posterior end with the inferior turbinate and perpendicular plate of palatine bone.

The ethmoid cells are divided into two groups: The anterior ethmoid cells, which lie anterior to the ground lamella of the middle turbinate and open in the middle meatus. The posterior ethmoid cells, which lie behind the ground lamella and open into the superior meatus or sphenoethmoidal recess. The ground lamella may be displaced anteriorly or posteriorly depending on the relative extent of pneumatization of the anterior or posterior ethmoidal air cells. The ethmoidal bulla is a large and fairly constant anterior ethmoid air cell . The ethmoidal cells are incomplete superiorly and posteriorly. They are completed superiorly by the frontal bone and posteriorly by the sphenoid bone. (Figs 2.10A and B). The ethmoid cells tend to migrate into the surrounding bones to develop variable patterns of pneumatization.

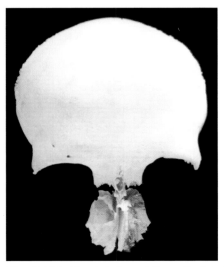

Fig. 2.10A: Frontal view of the articulated
frontal and ethmoid bones

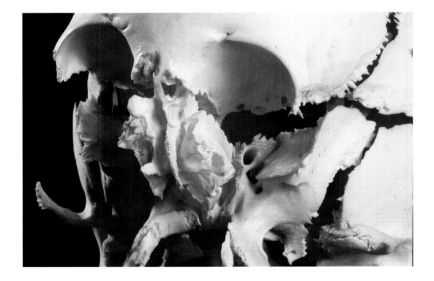

Fig. 2.10B: The articulated frontal, ethmoid and sphenoid bones

These paths of pneumatization include (see Figs 6.11A and B):

- Anterosuperiorly—into the frontal bone to form the frontal sinus.
- Superiorly—above the ethmoidal bulla over the orbit and behind the frontal sinus to form the supraorbital cell.
- Inferolaterally—into the roof of the maxillary sinus as the Haller cell.
- Posteriorly—above the sphenoid sinus as the Onodi cell.
- Anteriorly—into the lacrimal bone and frontonasal process of the maxilla as the agger nasi cells.
- Superiorly—into the frontal recess to form the different types of frontal cells.
- Isolated cells may be present within the ethmoid infundibulum. These are the infundibular cells (see Figs 3.12A and B).

The Sphenoid Bone (Figs 2.11A and B)

The sphenoid bone closes off the back of the nasal cavity and separates it from the anterior and middle cranial fossa. It is in relation with important structures

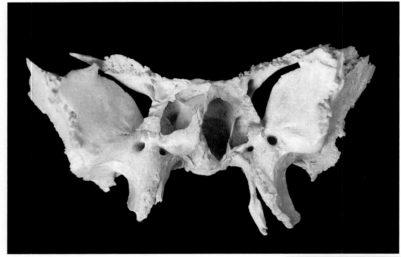

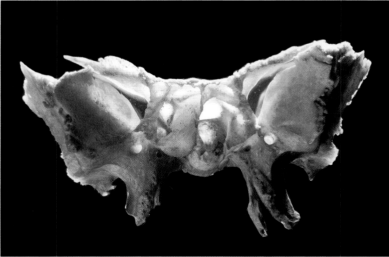

Figs 2.11A and B: Sphenoid bone

like the optic nerve and the carotid artery, making a good understanding of its anatomy very important to the operating surgeon.

Seen from the front, the sphenoid bone looks (with a little imagination!) like a bat with outstretched wings. The central portion is the body of the sphenoid, which is pneumatized by the two sphenoid sinuses. Anteriorly, in the midline is a strong triangular process called the rostrum, which articulates with the vomer.

Extending laterally from the central body on either side are a pair of greater wings and lesser wings. The retort-shaped superior orbital fissure lies between the greater and lesser wings. The lesser wing is attached to the body by two roots between which lies the optic canal. This canal transmits the optic nerve with its meninges and the ophthalmic artery. A stout process extends downwards on either side at the junction of the greater wing and the body of the sphenoid. This is the pterygoid process. It splits into the medial and lateral pterygoid plates. The medial pterygoid plate forms the lateral wall of the posterior choana. The lateral pterygoid plate is not in direct relation with the nasal cavity. The anterior surface of the pterygoid process forms the posterior wall of the pterygopalatine fossa. Two canals traverse the pterygoid process and present as foramina on its anterior surface. The inferomedial foramen is the funnel-shaped opening of the vidian canal for the vidian nerve. The supero-lateral foramen is the foramen rotundum, which transmits the maxillary nerve. It is important to note that the foramen rotundum lies just a few mms. below the superior orbital fissure.

The sphenoid sinuses are variably pneumatized. They are very often asymmetrical showing right- or left-sided *"sphenoidal dominance"*.

Depending on the pneumatization of the sphenoid bone, the sphenoid sinus can be classified into the following types (see Fig. 6.24):
- Conchal—a small pit-like depression.
- Presellar—extending up to the anterior wall of the pituitary fossa.
- Sellar—extending up to the clivus. The pituitary forms a distinct bulge in the roof of the sinus.
- Mixed.

The relations of the surrounding important structures are best understood in the sellar type. *Posterosuperiorly* in the midline of the roof lies the pituitary bulge. *Laterally* and *superiorly*, the optic canal can be visualized which at times is dehiscent. *Posteriorly* and *inferiorly*, the internal carotid artery bulge produces a prominence in the lateral wall. The sphenoid sinus may contain septae within it. These septae usually attach to important structures on the lateral wall of sphenoid sinus like the optic nerve or the internal carotid artery. A recess called the carotico-optic recess exists between the optic nerve and the internal carotid artery. This is especially deep when the anterior clinoid process is pneumatized, and the optic nerve may be dehiscent in such a case.

The Inferior Turbinate (Figs 2.12A and B)

The inferior turbinate is a separate scroll-like bone. Unlike the middle and superior turbinates, it runs a fairly straight course from anterior to posterior.

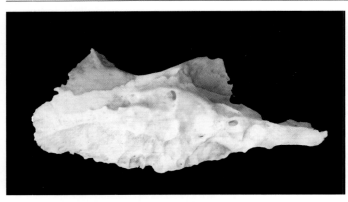 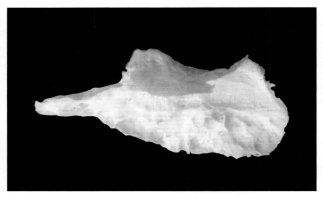

Figs 2.12A and B: (A) The right inferior turbinate (view on septal side): (1) lacrimal process (orange), (2) ethmoid process (blue), (B) The right inferior turbinate (view on meatal side) showing the maxillary process (green)

Its inferior margin is free and overhangs the inferior meatus. Its superior margin is attached to the maxilla anteriorly and the palatine bone posteriorly. Approximately, 1 cm behind its anterior end, its superior margin shows a peak or apex, which can be recognized in the live patient. The nasolacrimal duct opens into the inferior meatus at this peak.

The inferior turbinate has 3 processes:
1. Anteriorly, from its superior margin is the lacrimal process (it is this process, which forms the peak, mentioned earlier). The lacrimal process articulates with the descending process of the lacrimal bone and thus assists in forming the canal for the nasolacrimal duct.
2. A little behind the lacrimal process is another process arising from near the superior margin. This is the ethmoid process so called because it articulates with the uncinate process of the ethmoid bone. Thus, to recapitulate, the uncinate process is attached to the lacrimal bone at its anterior end and to the inferior turbinate posteriorly.
3. A third process arises from the superior border but curves laterally to attach to the maxilla. This is the maxillary process. It closes off part of the maxillary hiatus and forms part of the lateral wall of the inferior meatus.

Lacrimal Bone (Figs 2.13A and B)

The lacrimal bone is the smallest and most fragile of the cranial bones. It separates the orbit, more specifically the lacrimal fossa from the nasal cavity. The lacrimal bone articulates; *anteriorly* with the frontonasal process of the maxilla, *posteriorly* with the uncinate process, *superiorly* with the frontal bone and *inferiorly* it is drawn into a process called the descending process of the lacrimal bone. This, as we have discussed, articulates with the lacrimal process of the inferior turbinate to complete the medial wall of the nasolacrimal canal.

The orbital surface of the lacrimal bone has a crest, which is the posterior lacrimal crest (the anterior lacrimal crest is on the frontonasal process of the

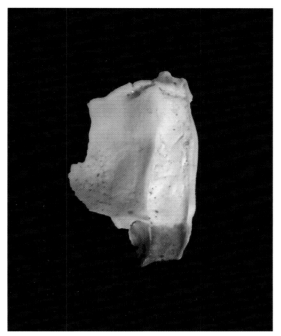 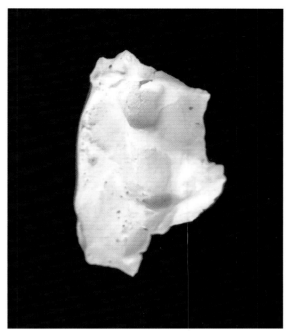

Figs 2.13A and B: The right lacrimal bone: (A) orbital surface, (B) nasal surface

maxilla). Between the two crests is the lacrimal fossa containing the lacrimal sac. The posterior lacrimal crest forms a hook inferiorly called the lacrimal hamulus. This forms the upper opening of the nasolacrimal duct. The nasal surface of the lacrimal bone is pneumatized by an anteriorly migrated ethmoidal cell, i.e. the agger nasi cell.

Palatine Bone (Fig. 2.14)

1. The palatine bone is a fragile L-shaped bone, which forms the posterior part of the lateral nasal wall and the floor of the nasal cavity. It consists of

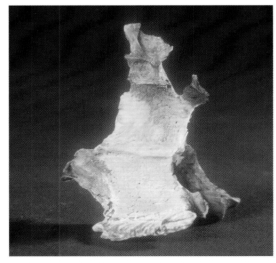

Fig. 2.14: The right palatine bone: (1) orbital process (orange), (2) sphenoidal process (green), (3) pyramidal process (magenta), (4) articulation with the inferior turbinate (purple)

two plates: a perpendicular plate, which forms the posterior part of the lateral nasal wall and the horizontal plate, which forms the posterior part of the nasal floor.

2. The perpendicular plate has a smooth medial surface, which is covered by nasal mucosa. This surface is divided into three sections by two crests running across it. The lower crest is called the conchal crest. The upper crest is called the ethmoidal crest. The conchal crest gives attachment to the inferior turbinate. The ethmoidal crest gives attachment to the middle turbinate. Thus, the area below the conchal crest forms part of the inferior meatus. The area between the two crests forms the posterior part of the middle meatus. Above the ethmoidal crest is a narrow groove, which forms part of the superior meatus. The sphenopalatine foramen opens into the nose just above the posterior attachment of the middle turbinate. It can, however, be approached through the middle meatus by detaching the middle turbinate from the ethmoidal crest.

3. The lateral surface of the perpendicular plate is smooth above and forms the medial wall of the pterygopalatine fossa. Inferiorly, the lateral surface is rough and articulates with the maxillary tuberosity. Between the two bones lies a canal for the greater palatine vessels and nerves.

   The palatine bone articulates with the surrounding bones in the following manner:

   Perpendicular plate
   - *The anterior border* of the perpendicular plate has a prolongation called the maxillary process. It articulates with the maxillary process of the inferior turbinate to close the maxillary hiatus.
   - *Posteriorly* with the medial pterygoid plates to form the lateral wall of the posterior choana.
   - *Inferiorly* it is continuous with the horizontal plate.
   - *Superiorly* with the maxilla by its orbital process and the sphenoid by its sphenoidal process.

   Horizontal plate
   - Anteriorly, it articulates with the horizontal process of the maxilla to form the nasal floor.
   - Posteriorly, it has a free border, which is the posterior end of the hard palate.

4. The palatine bone has three processes: two of these are at the superior border of the perpendicular plate. Of these, the anterior one is the orbital process, so called because it forms a small portion of the orbital floor near the posterior end of the inferior orbital fissure. The posterior process is the sphenoidal process, so called because it articulates with the body of the sphenoid. Between these two processes is a deep notch called the sphenopalatine notch. This is completed superiorly by the body of the sphenoid bone to form the sphenopalatine foramen. Thus, the spheno-palatine foramen gets its name from the fact that it lies between the sphenoid and the palatine bone. The third process is the pyramidal process, which extends posterolaterally from the junction of the perpendicular and horizontal plates. It articulates with the notch between the two pterygoid plates. It does not take part with the formation of the nasal cavity.

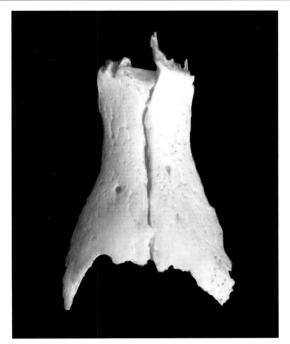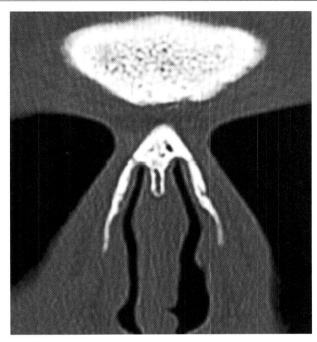

Figs 2.15A and B: Nasal bones

Nasal Bones (Figs 2.15A and B)

The nasal bones are two small rectangular bones, which form the bridge of the nose. They vary in size and form in different individuals. They have two surfaces and four borders:

- The external surface is covered by the procerus and nasalis muscle.
- The internal surface is concave from side to side. It has a groove for the anterior ethmoidal nerve.
- The superior border articulates with the frontal bone.
- The inferior border is related to the upper lateral cartilage.
- The lateral border articulates with the frontonasal process of the maxilla.
- The medial border widens into a vertical crest. It articulates with the opposite nasal bone and forms a small part of the septum of the nose.

The Lateral Nasal Wall

Dead men tell no tales........ but in our case they do!

3

The Lateral
Nasal Wall

Having studied the underlying osteology in the previous chapter, we will now re-articulate all the bones to form an intact lateral nasal wall and cover it with nasal mucosa. Thus due to the underlying bony processes and their articulation, the lateral nasal wall in the live person shows a series of elevations and depressions. We will study these in a sequential manner.

1. Anteriorly in the area of the nostril, the lateral nasal wall is lined by skin and has hair; this is the vestibule (Figs 3.1A and B). Behind this is a plain structureless area lined by nasal mucosa called the atrium. The atrium shows

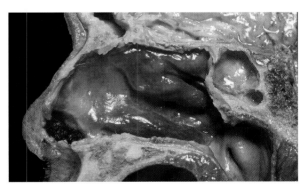
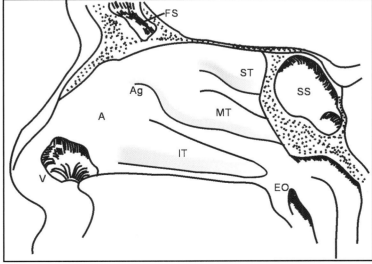

Figs 3.1A and B: The lateral nasal wall

a bulge anterior to the middle turbinate formed by the underlying agger nasi cell. Very often a ridge can be discerned extending from the agger nasi cell to an apex on the superior border of the inferior turbinate. This ridge overlies the nasolacrimal duct.

Behind the atrium are the three scrolls of the inferior, middle and superior turbinates, overlying the respective meatii. Occasionally, there may be a supreme turbinate. Above the superior turbinate is the sphenoethmoidal recess, which gets its name from the fact that this area forms a niche between the posterior ethmoid cells and the sphenoid sinus.

Certain other important features seen are:
- The inferior turbinate is fairly straight and structureless as compared to the middle turbinate, which is convoluted showing many features and anatomical variations.
- The posterior end of the middle turbinate ends at the level of the roof of the posterior choana.
- The eustachian tube lies in the nasopharynx at the level of the inferior turbinate 1 cm behind its posterior attachment. The fossa of Rosenmueller forms a deep cleft behind the torus tubaris.

A close up view of the skull base in the anterior cranial fossa shows (Fig. 3.2):
- The base skull sloping downwards from an anterior to posterior direction at an angle of 15°.
- The olfactory nerves can be seen perforating the cribriform plate.
- The frontal sinus is seen between the two tables of the frontal bone. Anteroinferior to the frontal sinus is the thickened frontal beak.
- The pituitary gland lies posterosuperior to the sphenoid sinus. The relationship of the pituitary and optic nerves to the sphenoid sinus is best seen in the well-pneumatized sellar type of sphenoid sinus. One can also see that the anterior wall of the sphenoid is thicker inferiorly than superiorly.

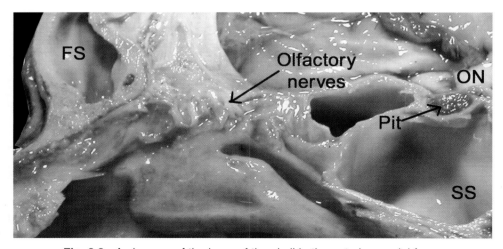

Fig. 3.2: A close up of the base of the skull in the anterior cranial fossa

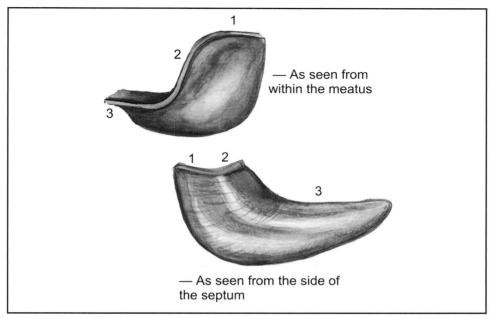

— As seen from
within the meatus

— As seen from the side of
the septum

Fig. 3.3: Attachments of middle turbinate (1) to cribriform plate and frontonasal process of the maxilla, (2) to lamina papyracea, (3) to perpendicular plate of palatine

2. The middle turbinate is a convoluted structure bending in different planes similar to a dried leaf. It can be divided into three parts, depending on its attachment and its orientation in the three-dimensional space (Fig. 3.3).
*   The anterior one-third is in the sagittal plane and is attached to the cribriform plate at the junction of the medial and lateral lamellae. It also takes a small anterior attachment to the frontonasal process of the maxilla.
*   The middle one-third lies in the coronal plane and is attached to the lamina papyracea. It separates the anterior ethmoidal cells from the posterior ethmoidal cells. Since it stabilizes the middle turbinate, it is called the ground lamella or the basal lamella.
*   The posterior third lies in the horizontal plane and is attached to the lamina papyracea and the perpendicular plate of the palatine bone extending upto the roof of the posterior choana.

3. A window is cut in the middle turbinate to view the relationship of structures within the middle meatus (Figs 3.4A and B). Most anteriorly is a curved ridge called the uncinate process. Behind this is the well pneumatized and most constant anterior ethmoidal cell, namely the ethmoidal bulla. These structures are separated by a semilunar groove called the hiatus semilunaris. The hiatus semilunaris is two-dimensional and leads into a three-dimensional space called the infundibulum.

The uncinate process, the bulla and the intervening infundibulum form the key area or the osteomeatal unit into which the frontal, the maxillary and anterior ethmoidal sinuses drain.

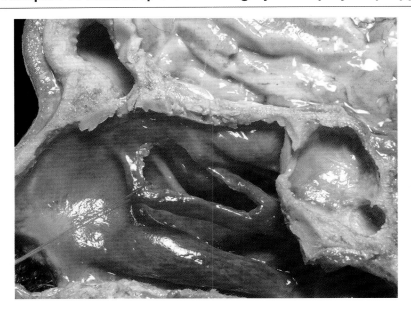

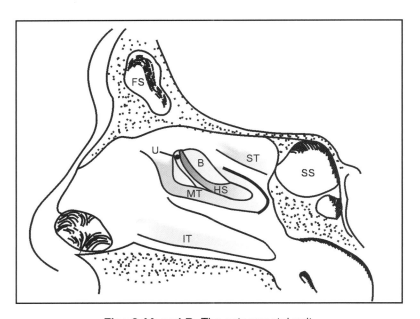

Figs 3.4A and B: The osteomeatal unit

Coronal and axial sections through the osteomeatal unit show the relationship between its components (Figs 3.5A and B).

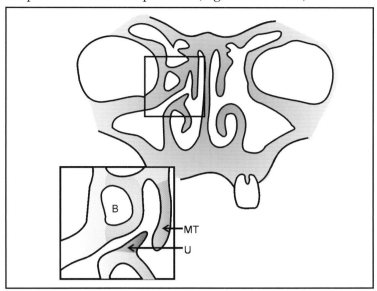

Fig. 3.5A: Coronal section of the osteomeatal unit

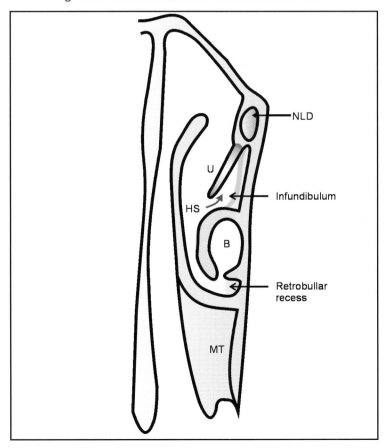

Fig. 3.5B: Axial section of the osteomeatal unit

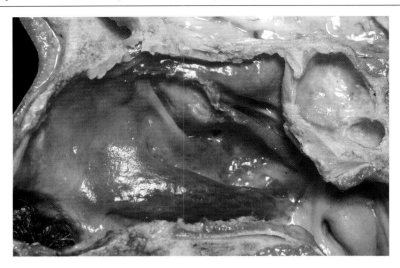

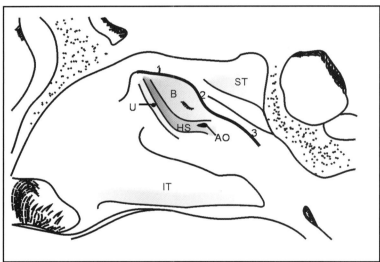

Figs 3.6 A and B: (1) Anterior attachment of middle turbinate to cribriform plate. (2) Middle attachment (ground lamella) to lamina papyracea. (3) Posterior attachment to perpendicular plate of palatine bone. An accessory ostium is seen in the hiatus semilunaris

4. The middle turbinate is trimmed. Its anterior, middle and posterior attachments, which have been described earlier are now obvious. The structures within the middle meatus are now seen more clearly (Figs 3.6A and B).

The uncinate process is sickle shaped. It has a vertical and a horizontal limb with an intermediate transitional part.

The ethmoidal bulla is usually a well pneumatized, most constant, anterior ethmoidal cell. Rarely (8%) the bulla may be rudimentary or absent. It is separated posteriorly from the ground lamella of the middle turbinate by a recess called the retrobullar recess (Fig. 3.7). Occasionally the bulla does not extend upto the base of the skull and is separated from it by the suprabullar recess. The retrobullar and suprabullar recesses together form a semilunar space

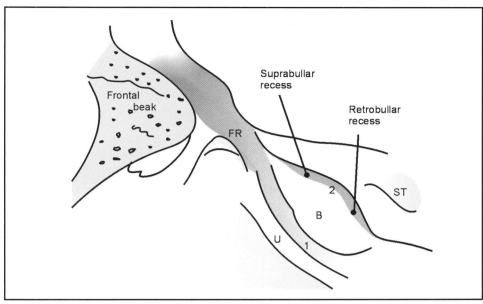

Fig. 3.7: The suprabullar and retrobullar recesses: (1) The hiatus
semilunaris inferoris, (2) the hiatus semilunaris superioris

above and behind the bulla called the sinus lateralis of Grunwald. This sinus opens into the middle meatus by a semilunar cleft which is opposite in orientation to the hiatus semilunaris and is called the hiatus semilunaris superioris. Thus the hiatus semilunaris inferioris leads into the infundibulum and the hiatus semilunaris superioris leads into the sinus lateralis of Grunwald.

The roof of the sinus lateralis is formed by the ethmoid fovea and its floor by the ethmoidal bulla. It is limited posteriorly by the ground lamella of the middle turbinate and anteriorly it opens into the frontal recess. Laterally is the lamina papyracea and medially is the middle turbinate. The hiatus semilunaris superioris is absent when the bulla is attached either to the base skull superiorly or to the ground lamella posteriorly.

5. The infundibulum leads directly or indirectly into the frontal recess (Figs 3.8A and B). The frontal recess has been the subject of many debates due to the fact that it shows variations in anatomy and requires special skill to approach it surgically.
- The frontal recess is bounded anteriorly by the agger nasi cell, which is considered to be a part of the frontal recess. Therefore the anterior wall of the frontal recess is formed by the anterior wall of the agger nasi cell.
- The posterior wall is formed by the bulla ethmoidalis. If there is a suprabullar recess it will open into the posterior wall of the frontal recess.
- The lateral wall of the frontal recess is formed by the lamina papyracea.
- The medial wall is formed by the middle turbinate.
- Superiorly the frontal recess opens via the frontal ostium into the frontal sinus. Seen from above the frontal sinus opening is funnel shaped and is placed at the posterior and medial end of the floor of the frontal sinus. This funnel shaped region is called the frontal infundibulum. Thus in sagittal

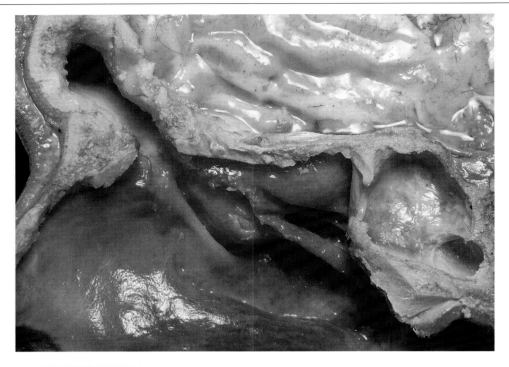

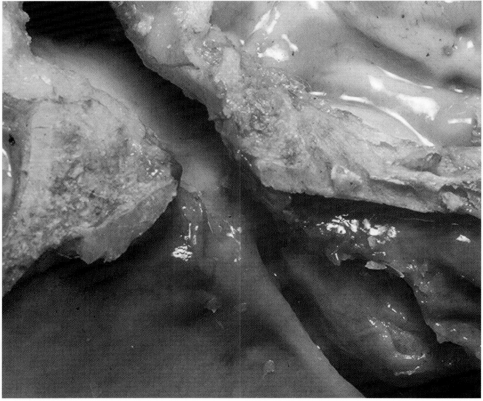

Figs 3.8A and B: (A) The frontal recess, (B) A close up view of
the frontal recess showing its boundaries and contents

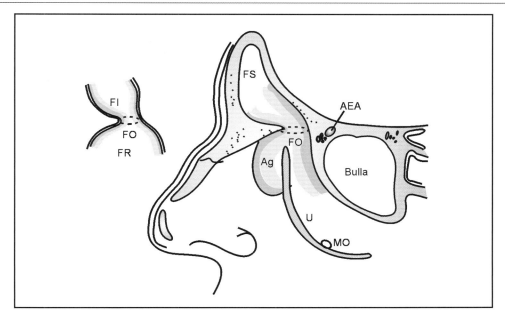

Fig. 3.9: Schematic representation of the frontal recess
(note the hour-glass configuration)

cross-section the frontal infundibulum, frontal ostium and the frontal recess together form the *"hour-glass configuration"* so often described (Fig. 3.9)

Thus, the frontal sinus lies far more anterior to the frontal recess when seen endoscopically.

The upper end of the uncinate process lies within the frontal recess. It shows great variation in anatomy. It can

— extend upto the base skull.
— attach to the middle turbinate.
— may turn forwards to be attached to the insertion of the middle turbinate.
— lie free in the middle meatus.
— may be pneumatized.

Most commonly (80%) it attaches to the lamina papyracea in the form of a dome. This upper dome shaped attachment of the uncinate process within the frontal recess has been graphically described by Stammberger as an eggshell in an inverted egg-cup. The recess, which is enclosed within this dome, is called the recessus terminalis (Figs 3.10A and B). In this case the frontal sinus opens medial to the uncinate process.

The components and contents of the frontal recess are extremely variable:

• The agger nasi cell may be small or large, single or multiple and rarely absent.
• The bulla may be small or large, extending upto base skull or stopping short at the suprabullar recess.
• The upper end of the attachment of the uncinate process has many variations, as already described.

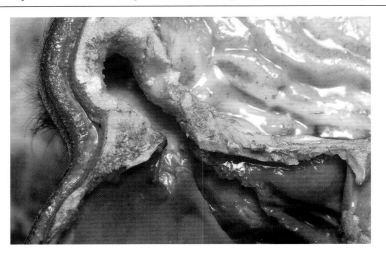

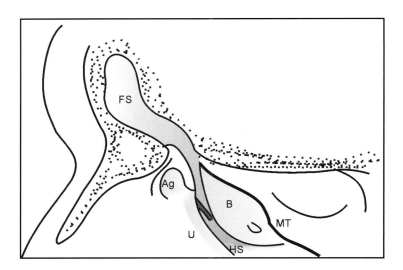

Fig. 3.10A and B: A blue probe inserted in the hiatus semilunaris cannot enter the frontal sinus as it is obstructed by the recessus terminalis

- The anterior ethmoidal cells may migrate anterosuperiorly into the frontal recess to produce different types of **frontal cells** viz

  Type I   A single cell above the agger nasi cell (Figs 3.11A and B).

  Type II   Two or more cells above the agger nasi cell.

  Type III   A large cell extending well into the frontal sinus mimicking the frontal sinus itself (frontal bulla).

  Type IV   An isolated **"loner cell"** separately within the frontal sinus.

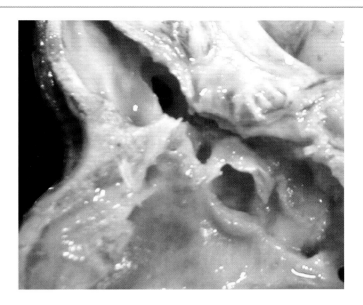

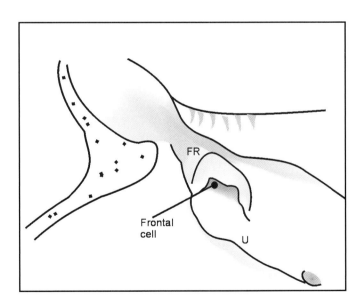

Figs 3.11A and B: The frontal recess showing a type I frontal cell

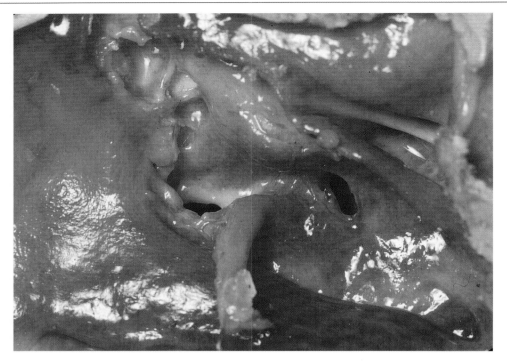

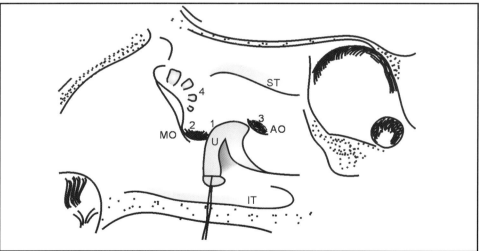

Figs 3.12A and B: The uncinate process is cut to reveal: (1) The infundibulum, (2) the maxillary ostium, (3) the accessory ostium, and (4) the infundibular cells

6. The uncinate process is cut to expose the infundibulum (Figs 3.12A and B). In the depths of the infundibulum, well hidden by the uncinate process lies the opening of the maxillary sinus. The normal ostium of the maxillary sinus is usually ovoid and tunnel like, having three-dimensions. Conversely the accessory ostium is easily seen, usually circular and has only two dimensions.

The relations of the maxillary ostium are: *Inferiorly* is the inferior turbinate, 1 to 2 mm *superiorly* is the lamina papyracea and the orbit, *posteriorly* is the posterior fontanelle, 0.5 cm *anteriorly* lies the nasolacrimal duct.

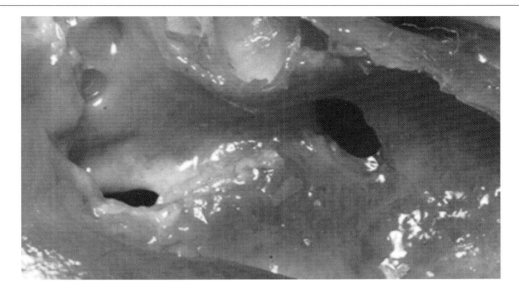

Fig. 3.12C: A close up view of normal and accessory maxillary ostia

The anterior fontanelle, an area of double layer of mucosa without any underlying bone, is found anteroinferior to the uncinate process (Fig. 3.12C). Similarly, the posterior fontanelle lies posterior and little above the posterior attachment of the uncinate process. The mucosa in these fontanelles may be dehiscent to produce accessory ostia.

7. The frontal recess, the maxillary sinus and the opening of the bulla into the middle meatus are visualized (Figs 3.13A and B). The bulla may drain into the middle meatus, the hiatus semilunaris inferioris or into the sinus lateralis when present. The frontal sinus drains into the frontal recess either medial or lateral to the uncinate process depending on the mode of attachment of the uncinate process. It may also drain into the suprabullar recess when it is present. The maxillary sinus shows no variation in drainage and always drains into the infundibulum. The sphenoid sinus drains into the sphenoethmoidal recess.

8. The anterior and posterior ethmoid cells are now dissected taking care to leave the anterior wall of the bulla and the ground lamella of the middle turbinate intact (Figs 3.14A and B). It can now be clearly seen that the endoscopic surgeon has to traverse four main barriers in the coronal plane as he proceeds deeper into the operative field.

These from anterior to posterior are—the uncinate process, the anterior wall of the bulla, the ground lamella and the anterior wall of the sphenoid. The surgeon may also encounter the ground lamella of the superior and if present the supreme turbinate if he dissects superolaterally.

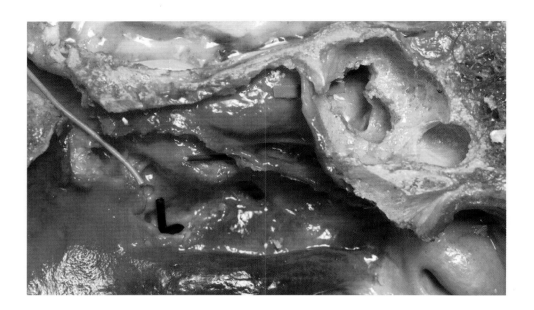

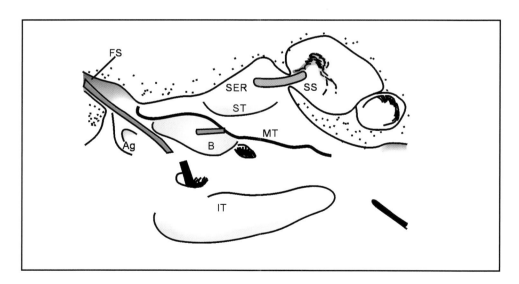

Figs 3.13A and B: Drainage of: (1) maxillary sinus (black), (2) bulla (blue),
(3) frontal sinus (light brown), (4) sphenoid sinus (green)

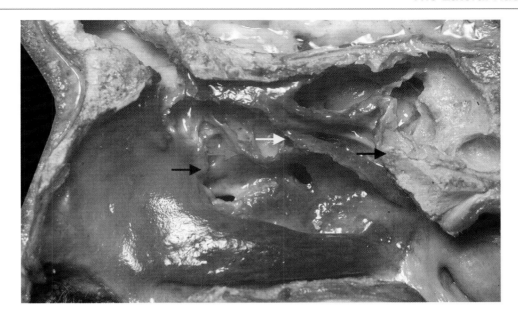

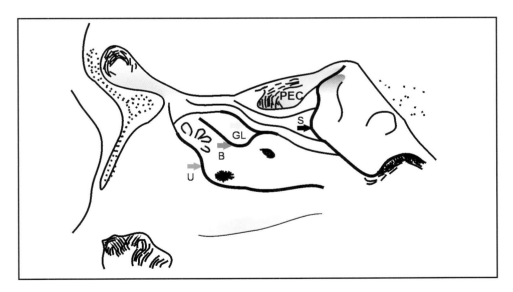

Figs 3.14A and B: Anterior and posterior ethmoidal cells dissected to show the four lamellae marked by arrows: (1) uncinate process (blue), (2) anterior wall of bulla (green), (3) ground lamella (yellow), (4) anterior wall of sphenoid (black)

9. The sphenoid sinus ostium lies high on its anterior wall close to its roof. It drains into the sphenoethmoidal recess. The superior turbinate in the spheno-ethmoidal recess, may over lie the opening of the sphenoid ostium. The anterior wall of the sphenoid sinus is thinner superiorly and thicker inferiorly where it forms the roof of the posterior choana. The sphenoid ostium lies 1-1.5 cm above the roof of the posterior choana and approximately 2-3 mm away from the septum.

One of the most important anatomical relationships that the endoscopic surgeon must understand is the relationship of the posterior ethmoid cells to the sphenoid sinus. Consider the following facts: in a sagittal section, the posterior ethmoidal cells can be seen extending for a short distance over the sphenoid sinus. They also lie in the lateral nasal wall compared to the sphenoid, which lies in the midline. The well-pneumatized sphenoid sinus extends posteriorly upto the clivus. Thus, the sphenoid sinus lies posterior, inferior and medial to the posterior ethmoid cells (Fig. 3.15A).

In 10 percent cases a posterior ethmoidal cell may extend posterolaterally over the sphenoid sinus for a much longer distance (Figs 3.15B and C). This cell is then called the Onodi cell. Thus the Onodi cell when present insinuates itself between the optic nerve and the sphenoid sinus. The optic nerve therefore produces a bulge in the Onodi cell instead of in the sphenoid sinus.

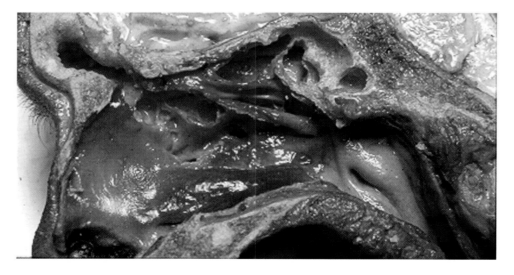

Fig. 3.15A: Relationship of the posterior ethmoid cells to the sphenoid sinus

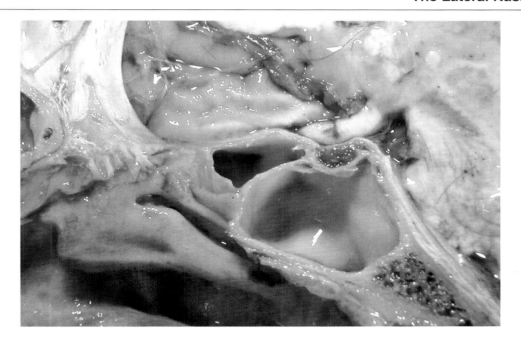

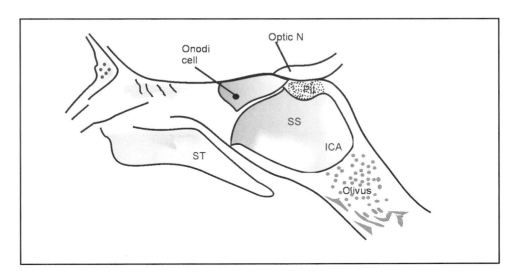

Figs 3.15B and C: The Onodi cell showing its relation
to the sphenoid sinus and the optic nerve

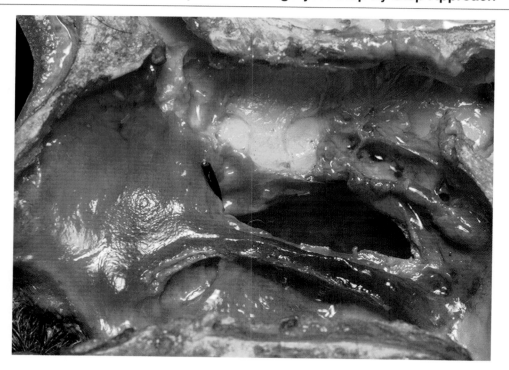

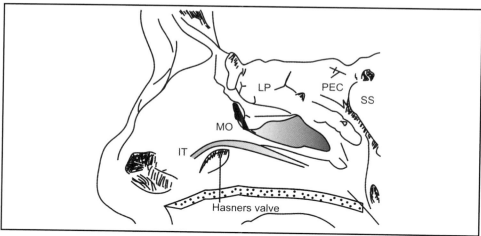

Figs 3.16A and B: The relationship of the maxillary ostium to the lamina papyracea

10. The ethmoidal cells have been completely cleared to expose the lamina papyracea, which appears yellowish due to the underlying orbital fat (Figs 3.16A and B). The maxillary ostium has been widened to gain a view of the interior of the sinus. It can be seen that the lamina papyracea and consequently the orbit is just 2-3 mm above the level of the maxillary ostium.

The inferior turbinate has been trimmed. It overlies a smooth fairly structureless inferior meatus. Although the inferior turbinate is fairly straight, its attachment shows a peak or apex approximately 1 cm behind its anterior

The Lateral Nasal Wall **49**

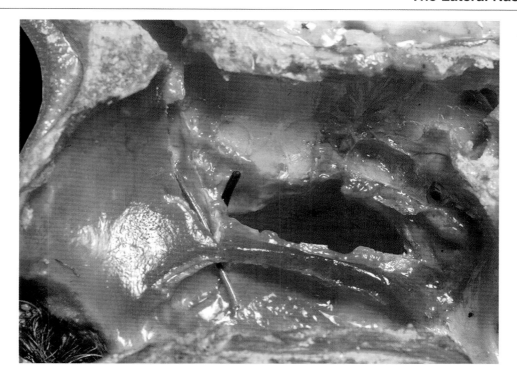

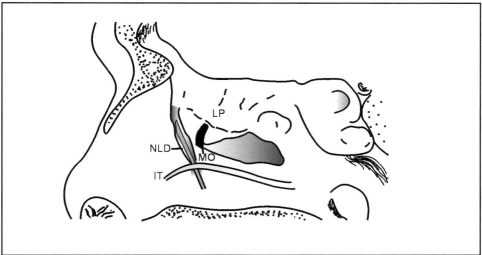

Figs 3.17A and B: Relationship of the maxillary ostium to the nasolacrimal duct

end (Figs 3.17A, B; 3.18A to C). The nasolacrimal duct opens in the roof of the inferior meatus at this apex. It is guarded by a valve called the Hasner's valve. The canal for the nasolacrimal duct has been dissected. It lies approximately 5 mm anterior to the normal maxillary ostium. The nasolacrimal duct is split open to visualize the lacrimal sac, the duct and the Hasner's valve.

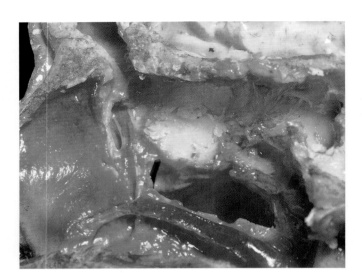

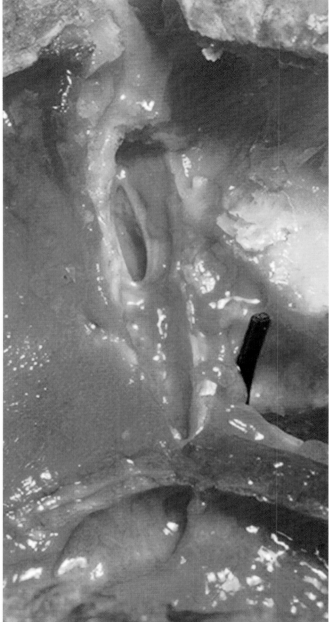

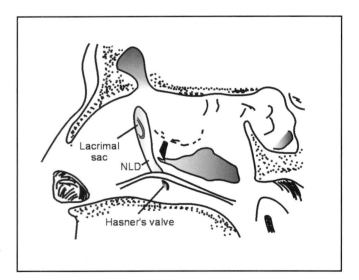

Figs 3.18A to C: The lacrimal apparatus and its close up

11. The lamina papyracea has been removed and the orbital periosteum has been cut to expose the orbital fat. Anteriorly, a pad of fat separates the vital structures of the orbit from the nose. However, posteriorly the medial rectus is in close relation with the lamina papyracea (Figs 3.19A to C).

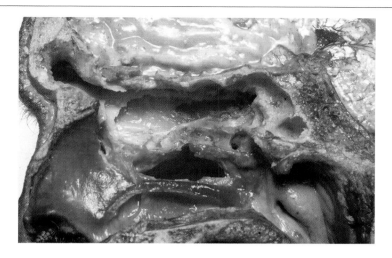

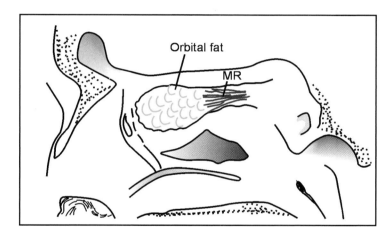

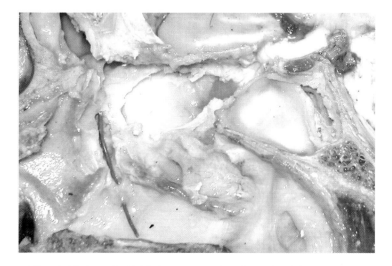

Figs 3.19 A to C: Orbital contents showing orbital fat anteriorly and medial rectus posteriorly

12. The medial rectus has been cut at the annulus of Zinn and reflected anteriorly. The intraconal compartment and the optic nerve can be seen (Figs 3.20A and B).

13. The sphenoid sinus is opened widely by removing the intersphenoid septum. There are two bulges in the lateral wall: *Superiorly* is the bulge of the optic nerve, *inferiorly* and *posteriorly* is the internal carotid artery. The groove between the two is the carotico-optic recess.

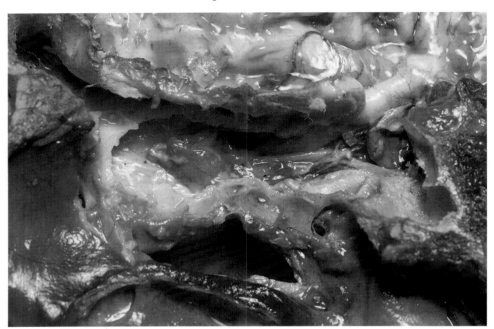

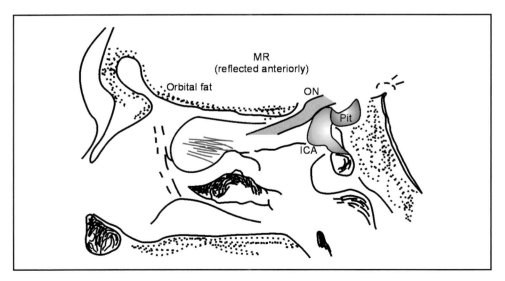

Figs 3.20A and B: Intraconal compartment of orbit—the medial rectus has been reflected anteriorly

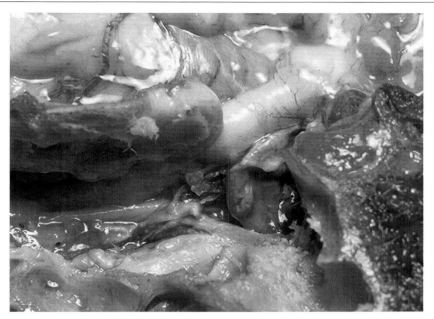

Fig. 3.20C: Close up view of Fig. 3.20A

An extensively pneumatized sphenoid sinus may show a lateral recess due to pneumatization of the greater wing between the foramen rotundum and the vidian canal. In such a case, two additional bulges can be seen: The maxillary nerve inferolaterally and the vidian nerve inferomedially.

The lateral wall of the sphenoid sinus has been dissected to expose the siphon of the internal carotid artery and the optic nerve. The relationships of the ICA, the optic nerve and the pituitary gland to each other can be seen (Figs 3.20A to D).

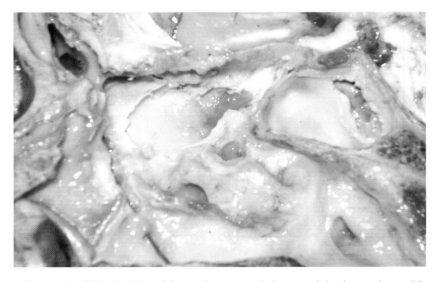

Fig. 3.20D: Relationship of the optic nerve, pituitary and the internal carotid artery to each other

Blood Supply of the Nose (Figs 3.21A and B)

Sr no. Artery	Branch of	Supplies
1. Anterior ethmoid 2. Posterior ethmoid	Ophthalmic artery (ICA)	Ethmoid and Frontal sinuses, roof of the nose, upper part of lateral wall and septum
3. Spheno-palatine	Maxillary artery (ECA)	Supplies the mucous membrane, superior and middle meatus, conchae and septum
4. Greater palatine	Maxillary artery (ECA)	• Posterior part of the lateral nasal wall as it decends in the greater palatine canal • Anterior inferior end of septum as it re-enters the nose through the incisive canal
5. Superior labial	Facial artery (ECA)	Region of the vestibule of the nose
6. Infraorbital 7. Posterior superior alveolar 8. Anterior superior alveolar	Maxillary artery (ECA)	Mucous membrane of the maxillary sinus
9. Pharyngeal branch	Maxillary artery (ECA)	Sphenoid sinus
10. Twigs from the internal carotid artery	—	Sphenoid sinus

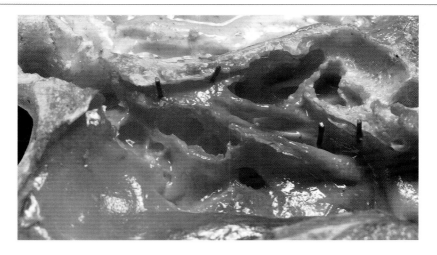

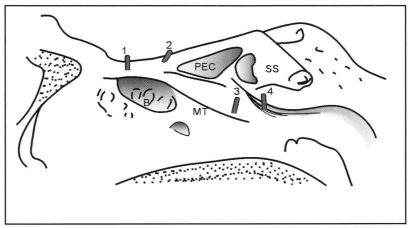

Figs 3.21A and B: Important vessels encountered: (1) Anterior ethmoid artery, (2) posterior ethmoid artery, (3) sphenopalatine artery, (4) septal branch of the sphenopalatine artery

Anterior Ethmoid Artery

The anterior ethmoid artery is given off from the ophthalmic artery in the orbit. It enters the nose, traverses across the roof of the ethmoidal sinus in an anteromedial direction and then leaves the nose at the lateral lamella of the cribriform plate to enter the cranial cavity. Thus the canal in which it traverses from the orbit to the cranial cavity is called the orbitocranial canal. The lateral end of the orbitocranial canal is at the suture line of the frontal bone and the lamina papyracea. The medial end of the canal at the cribriform plate is the thinnest part of the anterior cranial fossa. The canal is oblique and runs at a variable distance as much as 17 mm below the roof of the ethmoid to which it is attached by a bony mesentery. The anterior ethmoid artery lies 1-2 mm behind the point where the anterior wall of the bulla meets the base skull. If the bulla does not extend upto the base skull, the artery lies within the suprabullar recess. Another important endoscopic finding is that the artery is present where the vertical posterior wall of the frontal sinus turns to form the horizontal base skull.

On entering the cranial cavity the artery turns anteriorly along the cribriform plate in a sulcus called the ethmoidal sulcus. It gives off a meningeal branch and then re-enters the nasal cavity on either side of the crista galli. It then passes in a groove along the inner surface of the nasal bone supplying the upper part of the septum and the lateral nasal wall. It appears on the external surface of the nose through a notch between the nasal bone and the upper lateral cartilage.

Posterior Ethmoid Artery

The posterior ethmoid artery arises from the ophthalmic artery in the orbit and passes through the fissure between the frontal bone and the lamina papyracea 6 mm in front of the optic foramen to enter the nasal cavity. It usually lies high in the roof of the ethmoid and may not be easily seen. It passes anteromedially to gain entry into the cranial cavity at the level of the cribriform plate. It traverses the cribriform plate in an anterior direction for a short distance and passes through one of its foramina to re-enter the nasal cavity and supply the upper and posterior part of the nasal septum.

Sphenopalatine Artery

The sphenopalatine artery is the terminal part of the maxillary artery in the pterygopalatine fossa. It passes medially through the sphenopalatine foramen to enter the nasal cavity above the posterior end of the middle turbinate. It gives off lateral nasal branches, which supply the nasal conchae and meatii. Its medial branch crosses the anterior face of the sphenoid bone to supply the septum.

The sphenopalatine artery along with the terminal branches of the greater palatine artery, the anterior ethmoidal artery and the superior labial branch of the facial artery forms the Keisselbach's plexus in the Little's area, which is responsible for anterior epistaxis.

Endoscopic Anatomy

Begin by being a Surgeon on the dead body...
with as much care and precision as though it were a live
patient!

4

Endoscopic Anatomy*

Endoscopic anatomy is best studied using a fresh cadaver specimen, which has not being formalinized. This is because the feel of the tissues closely mimics that, which is felt during live surgery. However, in the absence of a fresh specimen, a formalinized cadaver will also reveal all the intricacies of anatomy to the avid learner. In learning endoscopic anatomy, we will try to follow the steps of surgery as closely as possible as in a live patient.

DIAGNOSTIC ENDOSCOPY

A careful and methodical diagnostic endoscopy is the key to understanding anatomical variations, pathological processes and to planning one's approach for surgery. It consists basically of three passes:

1st Pass

The 0° endoscope (or 30° endoscope) is passed gently along the floor of the nasal cavity between the inferior turbinate and septum without touching either structure (Fig. 4.1).

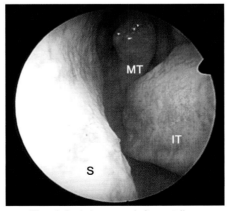

Fig. 4.1: 1st pass—left nostril

The septum is studied for any spurs and deviations. The inferior turbinate is examined for hypertrophy, especially at its posterior end. Any pathology obstructing the posterior choana is noticed (Fig. 4.2). The scope is advanced into the nasopharynx. The posterior wall and roof of the nasopharynx is examined to look for the presence of adenoids. The ipsilateral eustachian tube and the cleft behind it, i.e. the fossa of Rosenmueller, are examined (Fig. 4.3). The contralateral eustachian tube may also be seen but it is better seen with a 30° endoscope, which is advanced into the nasopharynx and rotated. The depths of the fossa of Rosenmueller are best studied by a 30° endoscope passed through the opposite nostril. On withdrawing the scope the inferior turbinate and septum are reviewed and the scope is rolled into the inferior meatus under the free margin of the inferior turbinate. As the scope is being withdrawn through the inferior meatus, the roof of the inferior meatus is

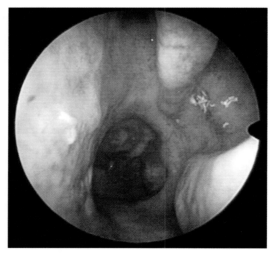

Fig. 4.2: 1st pass

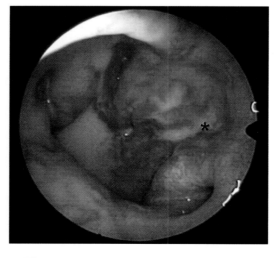

Fig. 4.3: 1st pass, fossa of Rosenmueller (∗)

studied for the opening of the nasolacrimal duct. This is guarded by a fold of mucous membrane called the Hasner's valve. This can be confirmed by the movement seen in this area on applying pressure near the lacrimal fossa. The scope is withdrawn out of the nostril.

2nd Pass (Figs 4.4A to C)

The scope is passed along the floor upto the posterior choana. It is then moved upward medial to the middle turbinate along the roof of the posterior choana and the anterior surface of the sphenoid. The superior turbinate and meatus are seen. The sphenoethmoidal recess is visualised. It lies between the superior turbinate laterally and the septum medially. It is bounded above by the base of the skull and is continuous inferiorly with the posterior part of the nasal cavity. The sphenoid ostium opens into the sphenoethmoidal recess 1-1.5 cm above the roof of the posterior choana and a few mms away fron the septum. It is very often hidden from view by the superior turbinate, which may need to be partially excised to visualize the ostium. The ostium shows variations in size and shape, being circular, oval and sometimes only pinpoint in configu-

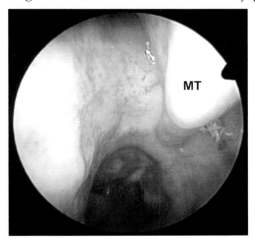

Fig. 4.4A: 2nd pass

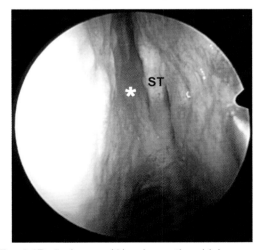

Fig. 4.4B: 2nd pass- (★) sphenoethmoidal recess

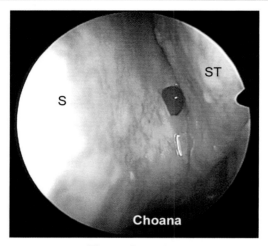

Fig. 4.4C: 2nd pass

ration. Below the ostium at the roof of the posterior choana is a mesh of blood vessels, which form the Woodruff's plexus. The septal branch of the sphenopalatine artery also runs across the anterior wall of the sphenoid in this region. This pass should be practiced as gently as possible without touching any of the turbinates as it can be quite painful in the live patient.

3rd Pass

The third pass is made to examine the contents of the middle meatus. The middle meatus can be entered by gently retracting the middle turbinate medially with the Freer's elevator. This may be difficult if the middle turbinate is rigid and may give rise to pain in the live patient.

The second simpler method to enter the middle meatus is to advance the scope posteriorly and roll the scope under the inferior border of the middle turbinate to enter the more roomy posterior part of the meatus. The scope is then withdrawn from posterior to anterior to view the contents of the middle meatus.

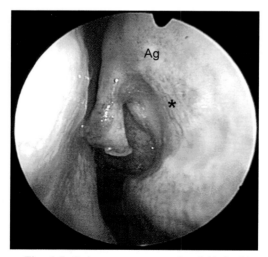

Fig. 4.5: 3rd pass, agger nasi cell (Ag), ridge
overlying nasolacrimal duct (∗)

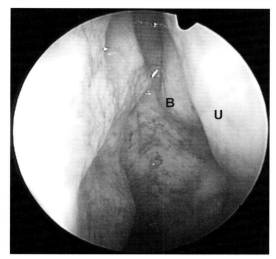

Fig. 4.6: 3rd pass

However, if one goes in an anterior to posterior direction one first sees the most anterior one-third attachment of the middle turbinate to the cribriform plate. This arch like attachment has also been called the axilla of the middle turbinate. The olfactory fossa can be examined in this area.

A bulge may be present in the region where the anterior end of the middle turbinate attaches to the lateral wall; this is formed by an underlying well-pneumatized agger nasi cell (Fig. 4.5). Within the meatus most anteriorly is the curved boomerang shaped uncinate process. A groove may be seen where the uncinate process attaches to the lateral wall. This is the junction of the uncinate process to the lacrimal bone. The area anterior to the uncinate process overlies the lacrimal sac. This area extends downwards in the form of a diffuse ridge to reach a "peak" in the attachment of the inferior turbinate. This ridge overlies the nasolacrimal duct. The bulge of the bulla is seen behind the uncinate process. The groove between the two i.e. the hiatus semilunaris is seen and palpated with a ballpoint, which enters the infundibulum (Fig. 4.6). A 30° scope can be used to inspect the infundibulum with a little manipulation. If the bulla does not reach the skull base the suprabullar recess is visualized and occasionally the anterior ethmoid artery can also be seen.

On retracting the middle turbinate gently, one can see that it turns laterally behind the bulla to attach to the lamina papyracea. This is the ground lamella.

As the scope is passed further posteriorly, the third or horizontal attachment of the middle turbinate is seen. It forms the roof of the middle meatus. The posterior end of the middle turbinate ends at the level of the roof of the posterior choana. Accessory ostia may be seen in the region of the anterior fontanelle, i.e. anteroinferior to the anterior end of the uncinate process, or in the posterior fontanelle i.e. above and behind the posterior end of the uncinate process. Accessory ostia are circular and are easily seen unlike the normal ostium, which can be ovoid, tunnel like and well hidden by the uncinate process (Fig. 4.7).

The middle turbinate may show different anatomical variations:
- Quite commonly it may be ballooned out due to an air cell enclosed within it. This air cell may be pneumatized from the frontal recess, agger nasi cell

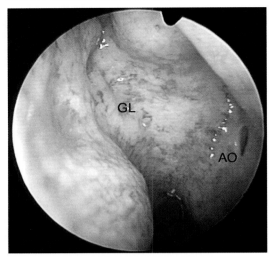

Fig. 4.7: 3rd pass

or anterior ethmoids. In such a case the middle turbinate is called the concha bullosa. This balloon like concha bullosa may block the osteomeatal unit and the drainage of the anterior group of sinuses.

- The vertical lamella of the middle turbinate may also be pneumatized from the superior meatus to form the interlamellar cell of Grunwald.
- The middle turbinate may have a paradoxical curve bending laterally towards the middle meatus.
- Occasionally, it may be bifid.
- The ground lamella of the middle turbinate may not attach to the lamina papyracea, but may miss the lamina papyracea, pass inferiorly to it and attach to the lateral wall of the maxillary sinus instead. The maxillary sinus in this case is divided into two parts. The posterior part behaves like a posterior ethmoidal cell because it drains behind the ground lamella of the middle turbinate (see Fig. 6.19).
- The lower part of a normally curved middle turbinate may curve far laterally to produce a concavity within it. This concavity is called the turbinate sinus (see Fig. 6.9).

The uncinate process is removed by a sickle knife or a backbiting forcep to expose the infundibulum (Fig. 4.8). The maxillary ostium can be seen lying in an oblique or horizontal plane behind the intermediate attachment of the uncinate process (Figs 4.9A and B). This can be widened posteriorly or anteroinferiorly to view the interior of the sinus with a 30° endoscope. The floor of the orbit and the infraorbital nerve can be visualized.

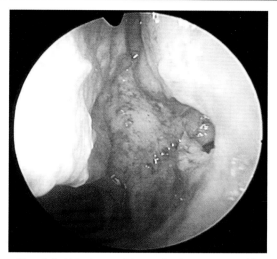

Fig. 4.8: Window cut in uncinate process with backbiting forceps

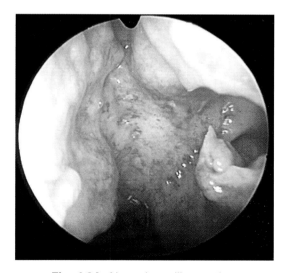

Fig. 4.9A: Normal maxillary ostium

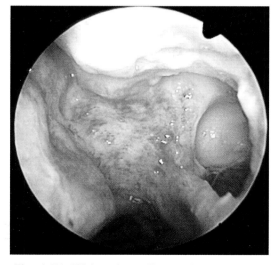

Fig. 4.9B: Widened maxillary ostium showing interior of maxillary sinus

The upper border of the attachment of uncinate process is removed along with any cells present in the frontal recess so as to expose the frontal sinus (Figs 4.10 to 4.13). The bulla is then perforated and is removed systematically in a lateral direction upto the lamina papyracea and in a superior direction upto the base skull. The posterior wall of the bulla is removed. The retrobullar and suprabullar recesses if present can be studied. The anterior ethmoidal artery may be seen running obliquely across the base skull. Occasionally the anterior ethmoid artery has a bony mesentery, which attaches it to the skull base.

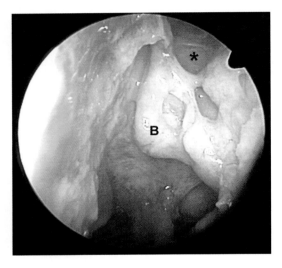

Fig. 4.10: Uncinate process removed. Bulla (B) and suprabullar recess (∗) seen

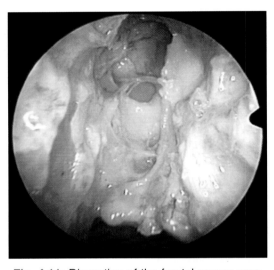

Fig. 4.11: Dissection of the frontal recess area

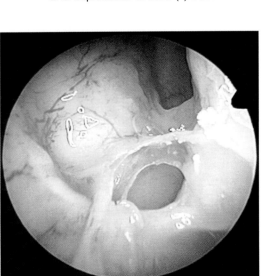

Fig. 4.12: Interior of frontal sinus

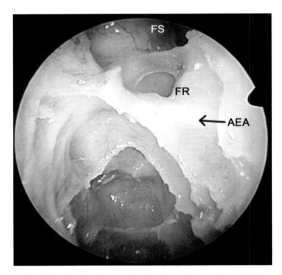

Fig. 4.13: The base skull after dissection of the frontal recess

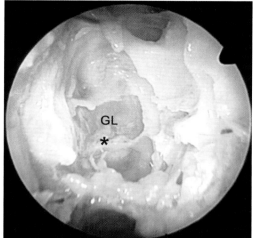

* → Entry point into posterior ethmoid cells

Fig. 4.14: The ground lamella

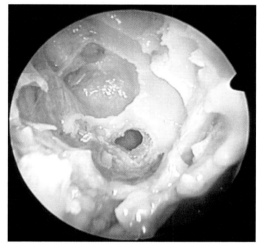

Fig. 4.15: Lateral approach to the sphenoid sinus—
posterior ethmoid cells have been removed

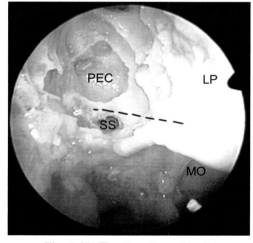

Fig. 4.16: The "maxillary ridge"

The ground lamella is then visualized (Fig. 4.14). Its position is confirmed by following the middle turbinate backwards to the point where it turns laterally. The ground lamella is perforated inferomedially to enter the posterior ethmoid cells. Care should be taken to preserve the inferior border of the ground lamella, so as to maintain the stability of the middle turbinate. The posterior ethmoid cells are larger in size as compared to the anterior ethmoid cells. They are removed completely to expose the lamina papyracea laterally, the base skull superiorly and the superior turbinate medially. The posterior most ethmoidal cell has a pyramidal shape, which tapers to a point posteriorly. The posterior ethmoidal artery may be seen running across the base skull. The sphenoid is opened inferomedially (Fig. 4.15). It is important to note that the bony partition dividing the posterior ethmoids from the sphenoid is not in a coronal plane but in an oblique or almost axial plane. The sphenoid sinus appears globular like the inside of a rounded pot as opposed to the pyramidal shape of the posterior most ethmoid cell. Another landmark is the "maxillary ridge". This ridge is an imaginary line between the medial and inferior wall of the orbit and extends backwards from the upper border of the maxillary ostium. If this ridge is extrapolated backwards then those cells which open above the level of this ridge are the posterior ethmoid cells. The cell, which opens below the level of this ridge, is usually the sphenoid sinus (Fig. 4.16).

The sphenoid sinus is opened widely to examine its walls (Fig. 4.17A). The lateral wall shows a bulge superiorly which is the optic nerve, below and slightly behind is the bulge of the internal carotid artery. There is a recess, which separates these two structures called the carotico-optic recess. This recess may be very deep if the anterior clinoid process is pneumatized. In a well-pneumatized sphenoid, the bulge of the pituitary may be seen posterosuperiorly in the midline. The intersphenoid septum may not be in the midline leading to unequal sphenoid sinuses or a "dominance" of one sphenoid sinus. Intra-sphenoid septae may be present and these usually attach to vital structures like the optic nerve and the carotid artery (Fig. 4.17B). Dehiscence of the optic nerve or internal carotid artery may be noticed. The surgeon must take care whilst removing polyps from within the sphenoid sinus and also whilst removing septae within the sphenoid sinus.

Occasionally an Onodi cell may grow above the sphenoid sinus, in which case, the optic nerve may be seen in its lateral wall.

The sphenoid sinus can be approached medial to the middle turbinate (Fig. 4.18). The sphenoid ostium is visualized and the anterior wall of the sphenoid is punched downwards to open the sphenoid sinus.

The sphenoid sinus may also be approached by an intermediate route. One can go through the posterior end of the middle turbinate to gain access to the sphenoethmoidal recess and the normal sphenoid ostium, which can then be widened.

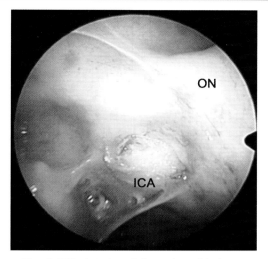

Fig. 4.17A: Interior of the sphenoid sinus

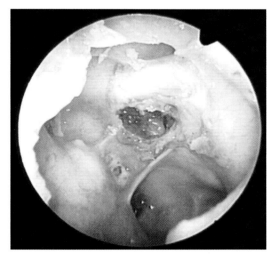

Fig. 4.17B: Intrasphenoid septae
attaching to ICA

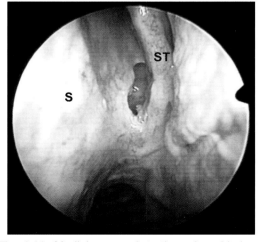

Fig. 4.18: Medial approach to the sphenoid sinus

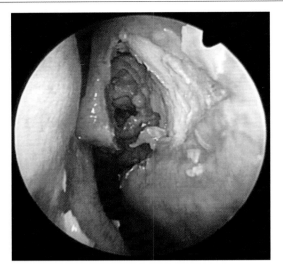

Fig. 4.19A: Dissection of nasolacrimal
apparatus —mucosal flap elevated

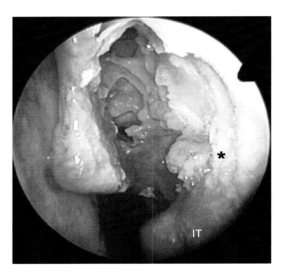

Fig. 4.19B: Bone removed to expose the
lacrimal apparatus, nasolacrimal duct (★)

The mucosa over the lacrimal bone can be removed (Figs 4.19A and B).
Suture lines can be seen separating the lacrimal bone from the uncinate process
posteriorly and from the frontonasal process of the maxilla anteriorly. The
lacrimal bone is removed to expose the lacrimal sac and dissection can be carried
out inferiorly to view the nasolacrimal duct.

Radiological Anatomy

*"Don't just do something...
Stand there and think!!!"*
— Ron Hoille

5

Radiological Anatomy

Safe, meticulous and complete endoscopic surgery can only be performed by a surgeon who has a sound knowledge in interpreting CT scans of the paranasal sinuses. The traditional X-rays of the paranasal sinuses are all but redundant for two reasons. Firstly, the diagnosis of acute or chronic sinusitis is a clinical one. Secondly, if surgical intervention is required in either of these cases, then the information gained from an X-ray paranasal sinus is too inadequate and a CT scan becomes mandatory.

The CT scan is the gold standard investigation in all preoperative cases and cannot be replaced by the MRI because it gives detailed bony anatomy of the area and serves as a "road map" for the operating surgeon. CT scans are best done after a course of antibiotics, so that acute inflammation is not mistaken for chronic mucosal disease. It is also advisable to ask the patient to blow his nose to clear out loose secretions prior to the CT scan. One should study the scout film provided by the radiologist first (Figs 5.1A and B).

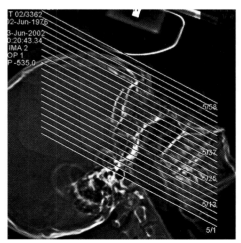

Fig. 5.1A: Scout film—3 mm slice thickness

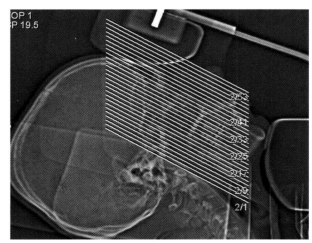

Fig. 5.1B: Scout film—1 mm slice thickness

Most of the anatomical details can be seen well in coronal sections. However, certain structures, e.g. the pterygopalatine fossa, fossa of Rosenmueller and the optic nerve are better seen on axial scans. A sagittal reconstruction allows us to study the anatomy of the lateral nasal wall and is especially useful to study the region of the frontal recess. Patients with dental fillings show many artefacts in coronal sections. In such cases, axial films can be taken and coronal reconstructions obtained. A very basic paranasal sinus study would include bony and soft tissue windows of 3 mm cuts taken anterior to posterior in the coronal plane. However, certain cases, e.g. optic nerve injury or CSF rhinorrhea would require 1 mm cuts for adequate evaluation. The coronal sections are routinely read from anterior to posterior and the axial sections from inferior to superior.

Coronal Scans

• The most anterior cuts show the frontal sinus and the nasal bones (Fig. 5.2A). The frontal sinus shows great variation in pneumatization. The interfrontal sinus septum is in the midline inferiorly but may deviate to either side of the midline as it goes posterosuperiorly to attach to the posterior wall of the frontal sinus. The interfrontal sinus septum may at times be pneumatized. Septae within the frontal sinus may lead to the formation of deep lateral recesses. The multiple frontal septae show a classical scalloping of the frontal sinus, which is lost in cases of mucoceles (Fig. 5.2B).

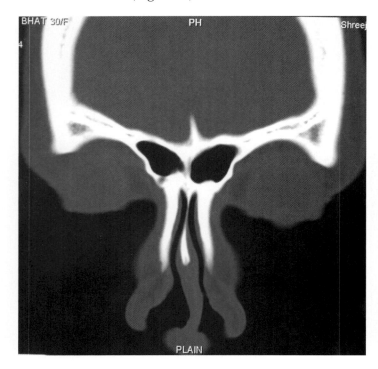

Fig. 5.2A: Anterior cut showing frontal sinus and nasal bones

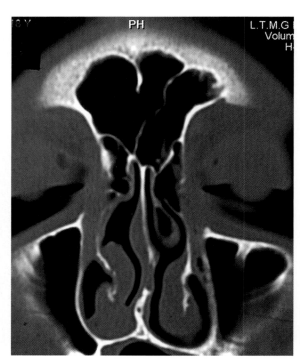

Fig. 5.2B: Cut showing interfrontal septum, scalloping of frontal sinus

- The inferior turbinate is visualized, any hypertrophy of the inferior turbinate is looked for. A mucosal swelling is seen in the anterior part of the septum. This is the septal tubercle, which consists of erectile tissue and is the phylogenetic remnant of the vomeronasal organ. The septum should be studied for deviations and septal spurs (Fig. 5.3).

- The middle turbinate is not yet seen. The air cells in this region are the agger nasi cells. The nasolacrimal duct is visualized. The presence of frontal cells, type I to IV should be looked for (Fig. 5.4).

- The middle turbinate is visualized; any anatomical variations like the concha bullosa or a paradoxically curved middle turbinate should be looked for.

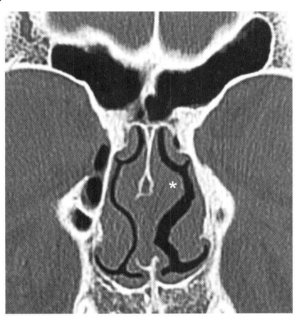

Fig. 5.3: The septal tubercle(∗)

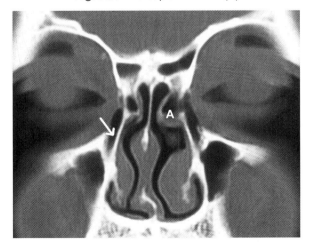

Fig. 5.4: Agger nasi cells (A), nasolacrimal duct (arrow), middle turbinate not yet visualized

- The attachment of the middle turbinate at the junction of the medial and lateral lamellae of the cribriform plate is seen (Fig. 5.5). The level of the cribriform plate and the depth of the olfactory fossa should be assessed and classified according to the Keros classification. The height of the ethmoidal fovea above the level of the cribriform plate is noted. Pneumatization of the crista galli may be visualized.

- The ethmoidal bulla is seen lateral to the middle turbinate. If the ethmoidal bulla does not extend to the skull base, the suprabullar recess may be visualized. A cell extending above the orbit, behind the frontal sinus may be seen in this cut. This is the supraorbital cell, which drains into the suprabullar recess (Fig. 5.6).

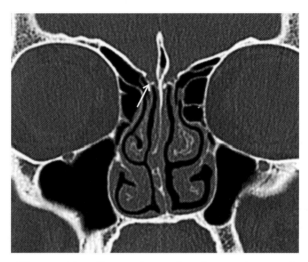

Fig. 5.5: The olfactory fossa. Anterior attachment of middle turbinate seen (arrow)

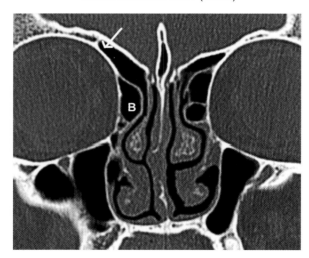

Fig. 5.6: The ethmoidal bulla and supraorbital cell (arrow)

- The uncinate process is seen below the bulla (Figs 5.7A and B). The groove between the uncinate process and the bulla, i.e. the hiatus semilunaris and the infundibulum are seen leading into the normal maxillary ostium. This is the osteomeatal unit.

- It should be noted whether any of the septal spurs impinge upon, or compromise the osteomeatal unit. Hypertrophy of the turbinates or a concha bullosa on the side opposite to the septal deviations should be looked for.

- The mode of attachment of the uncinate process should be carefully studied so as to ascertain the pathway of drainage of frontal sinus (Fig. 5.8). Variations in the anatomy of the uncinate process, and the presence of Haller cells should be looked for.

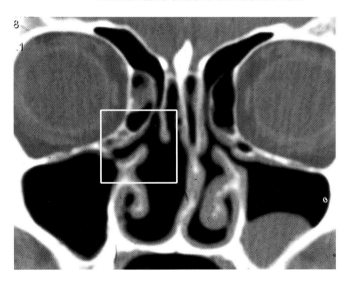

Fig. 5.7A: Osteomeatal unit

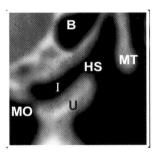

Fig. 5.7B: Osteomeatal unit (close up view)

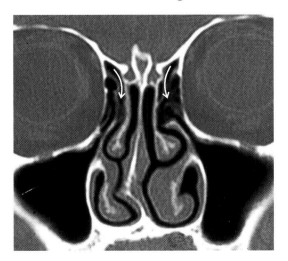

Fig. 5.8: Drainage of frontal recess—medial to infundibulum on the right and into the infundibulum on the left

- Accessory ostia may be seen in the region of the anterior and posterior fontanelle (Fig. 5.9).

- The maxillary sinus is seen. It is triangular in shape in this section. The infraorbital nerve is seen in the roof of the maxillary sinus (Fig. 5.10). At times it may be dehiscent.

- 2-3 mm behind the bulla, the anterior ethmoidal artery is seen as a classical *"beaking"* of the medial orbital wall (Fig. 5.11). The artery may lie close to the skull base or may cross low within the anterior ethmoids in which case the orbitocranial canal with its bony mesentery is clearly seen.

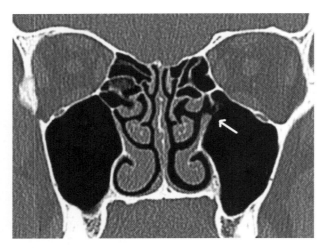

Fig. 5.9: Accessory ostium in the left posterior fontanelle

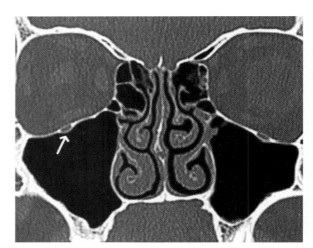

Fig. 5.10: Maxillary sinus appears triangular in anterior cuts (arrow: infraorbital nerve)

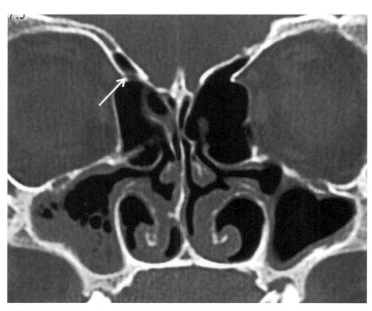

Fig. 5.11: Anterior ethmoidal artery. Beaking of lamina papyracea seen on left. Orbitocranial canal seen on the right (arrow)

- The middle turbinate is attached to the lamina papyracea by its ground lamella (Fig. 5.12A). This lamella is seen separating the anterior ethmoid cells from the posterior ethmoid cells. The superior turbinate is visualized in the more posterior cuts and any variations in it, e.g. pneumatization, paradoxical curvature should be looked for. The posterior most attachment of the middle turbinate to the palatine bone is seen (Fig. 5.12B).

- The posterior ethmoid cells are larger and fewer than the anterior ethmoid cells. The posterior ethmoid artery may occasionally be identified in the region of the skull base. The maxillary sinus changes shape from triangular to ovoid, in more posterior cuts. The orbit changes from a circular outline to a triangular or pyramidal shape. The posterior part of the orbit with the extraocular muscles and the optic nerve is seen. The fissure between the orbit and the maxillary sinus, i.e. the inferior orbital fissure is seen in this section. The infraorbital fissure opens laterally into the infratemporal fossa (Fig. 5.13). It is important to know that the medial rectus is separated from

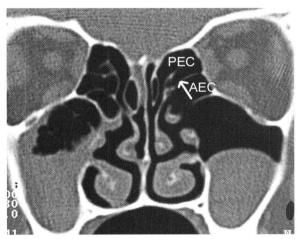

Fig. 5.12A: The ground lamella (arrow). Intermediate attachment of middle turbinate

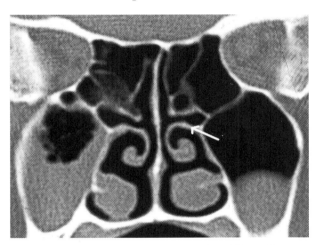

Fig. 5.12B: Posterior attachment of middle turbinate

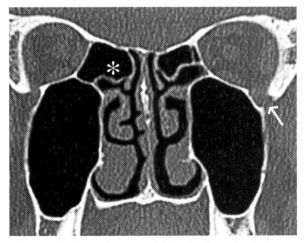

Fig. 5.13: Posterior ethmoidal cells (asterix). Inferior orbital fissure (arrow)

the lamina papyracea by a pad of fat anteriorly. However, more posteriorly in the orbit this pad of fat is absent and the medial rectus is in direct relation to the lamina papyracea and therefore more prone to injury (Figs 5.14A and B).

- The sphenoid sinus is seen. In the more anterior cuts both the posterior ethmoid cells and the sphenoid sinus are seen. The superolateral cell is the posterior ethmoid cell whereas the inferomedial cell is the sphenoid sinus. The more subsequent cuts show the sphenoid anatomy more clearly. The sphenoid dominance should be noted when the intersphenoid septum is asymmetrical. The sphenoid sinus ostium may also be visualized though this is better seen in sagittal cuts (Fig. 5.15). Accessory septae within the sphenoid should be looked for and traced to see if they are attached to

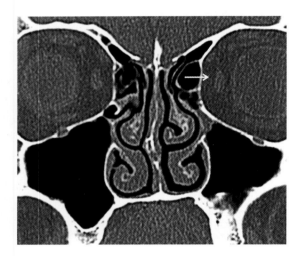

Fig. 5.14A: Fat intervening between lamina papyracea and medial rectus anteriorly

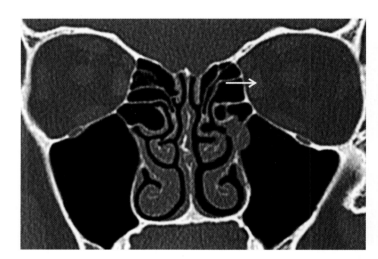

Fig. 5.14B: Medial rectus in direct contact with lamina papyracea posteriorly

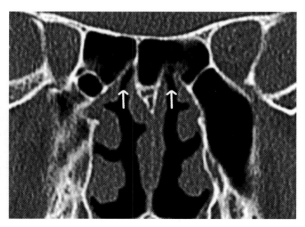

Fig. 5.15: Bilateral sphenoid ostia

vital structures. The optic nerve and the internal carotid artery are studied for any dehiscence of the overlying bone. Pneumatization of the anterior clinoid process leading to an almost bare optic nerve protruding into the sphenoid sinus should be looked for. In the presence of an Onodi cell superolateral to the sphenoid sinus, special attention should be paid to the course of the optic nerve. The extent to which the pituitary bulges into the sphenoid sinus will depend on the extent of pneumatization. This is best appreciated in sagittal reconstructions.

- The retort-shaped orbital apex is seen on either side of the sphenoid sinus in the anterior cuts (Figs 5.16 and 5.17). The pterygoid processes extend downwards and are perforated by two canals. The first is the foramen rotundum, which is seen just below the orbital apex. Inferomedial to this

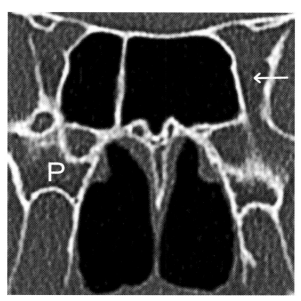

Fig. 5.16: Orbital apex (arrow), sphenoid dominance (left), pterygoid processes (P)

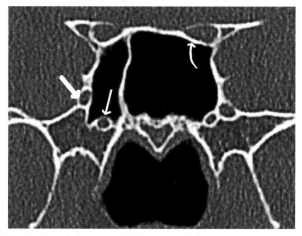

Fig. 5.17: Vidian canal (thin arrow), foramen rotundum (thick arrow), and optic nerve (curved arrow)

foramen is the opening of the vidian canal. The pterygoid processes form the posterior wall of the pterygopalatine fossa (the pterygopalatine fossa itself is best seen in axial sections). A canal may be seen below the sphenoid sinus between the pterygopalatine fossa and the posterior choana (Fig. 5.18). This is the sphenopalatine foramen, which opens above the posterior end of the middle turbinate. The sphenoid sinus may extensively pneumatize the pterygoid process and the greater wing of sphenoid to produce a large lateral recess extending between the foramen rotundum and vidian canal.

- Coronal sections of the nasopharynx show the eustachian tube opening, the torus tubaris, the fossa of Rosenmueller and the adenoids, if present (Fig. 5.19). Asymmetry of the fossa of Rosenmueller should be looked for. The foramen ovale is seen laterally in the greater wing of sphenoid (Fig. 5.20). Widening or destruction of the foramen should be looked for in a case of nasopharyngeal angiofibroma or a carcinoma of nasopharynx respectively.

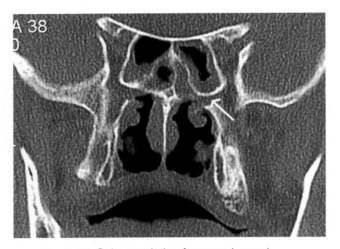

Fig. 5.18: Sphenopalatine foramen (arrow)

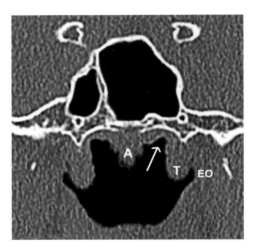

Fig. 5.19: Torus tubaris (T), fossa of Rosenmueller (arrow), adenoids (A)

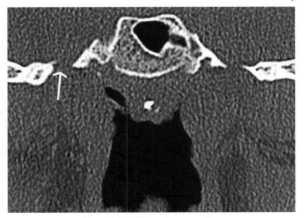

Fig. 5.20: Foramen ovale

Axial Scans

Certain structures are well seen on axial cuts:

- The nasolacrimal duct is seen as a circular opening at the anteromedial corner of the maxillary sinus (Fig. 5.21). Its anterolateral walls are thick, whereas its medial wall is comparatively thinner.
- Anteroposterior deviations of the septum can be assessed.
- The nasopharynx can be studied well in axial cuts and asymmetry of the fossa of Rosenmueller can be looked for (Fig. 5.22).
- An axial section through the middle turbinate will show its ground lamella and its attachment to the lamina papyracea (Figs 5.23A and B). The anterior ethmoid cells can be demarcated from the posterior ethmoid cells on the basis of this ground lamella. The space between the bulla and the ground lamella, i.e. the retrobullar recess when present can also be seen in axial sections.

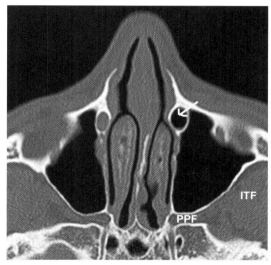

Fig. 5.21: Nasolacrimal duct (arrow)

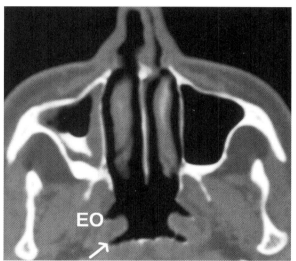

Fig. 5.22: Fossa of Rosenmueller (arrow), EO—eustachian tube opening

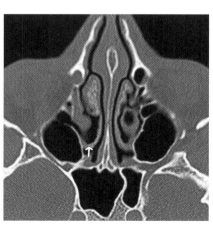

Fig. 5.23A: The ground lamella (arrow)

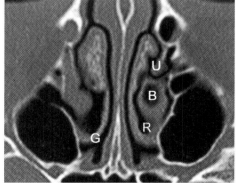

Fig. 5.23B: G: ground lamella, B: bulla, R: retrobullar recess, U: uncinate process (close up view)

- The maxillary sinus, the medial and lateral pterygoid plates and the intervening pterygopalatine fossa can be seen (Fig. 5.21). The pterygopalatine fossa opens medially into the nose via the sphenopalatine foramen. Laterally, it opens into the infratemporal fossa. The anterior, posterolateral and medial walls of the maxillary sinus can all be studied in the axial cuts. The roof and the floor of the maxillary sinus are better studied in coronal cuts.
- The lamina papyracea runs a fairly straight course in an anteroposterior direction (Fig. 5.24). However, in lower cuts of the orbit the upper part of the maxillary sinus is also seen; and hence, the lamina papyracea appears to take an abrupt curve laterally into the orbit (Fig. 5.25). Any natural dehiscence in the lamina should be looked for.
- Axial sections give an excellent opportunity to study structures in the orbit, i.e. the medial and lateral rectus, the intraconal, the extraconal and preseptal compartments (Fig. 5.24). The optic nerve can be traced in its entire course and its relation to a pneumatized anterior clinoid process or Onodi cell can be ascertained.

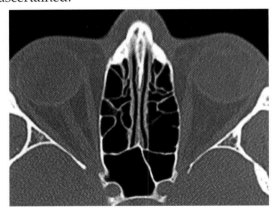

Fig. 5.24: The orbit in axial section

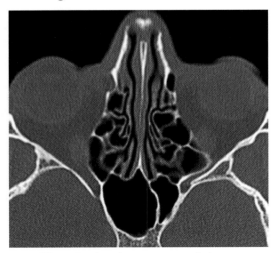

Fig. 5.25: Lamina papyracea in lower
section of the orbit

- The sphenoid sinus can be examined for asymmetry. Dehiscence over the internal carotid artery is better appreciated in axial cuts than in coronal cuts.
- The cavernous sinus can be seen on either side of the sphenoid sinus. It is better studied after injection of contrast.
- The cribriform plate, crista galli and foramen caecum can be studied in 1 mm sections (Fig. 5.26). Anterior to the cribriform plate is the frontal sinus. The anterior and posterior walls of the frontal sinus are better appreciated in axial than in coronal sections.

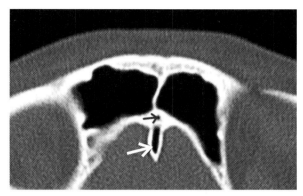

Fig. 5.26: Crista galli (thick arrow), foramen cecum (thin arrow)

Sagittal Sections

The sagittally reconstructed section gives an excellent opportunity to study details of the lateral nasal wall anatomy (Figs 5.27A and B).

- The four lamellae that the endoscopic surgeon has to cross in an antero-posterior direction are well seen in a single cut on the sagittal section. The

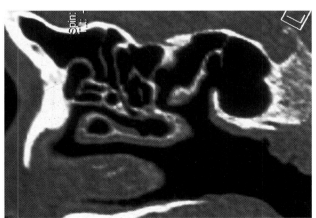
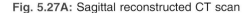

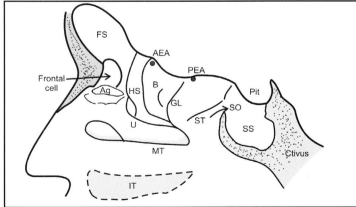

Fig. 5.27A: Sagittal reconstructed CT scan

Fig. 5.27B: Schematic representation of the sagittal CT scan

anterior and posterior ethmoids and sphenoid sinus are well demarcated from each other on the basis of these lamellae.

- The retrobullar and suprabullar recesses (sinus lateralis) if present, can also be seen.
- It is especially useful to study anatomy of the frontal recess area and should be asked for prior to operations on the frontal sinus.
- Pneumatization of the sphenoid in relation to the pituitary fossa can also be studied prior to pituitary surgery. The sphenoid sinus ostium is also better seen on sagittal cuts.
- The extent to which an Onodi cell has migrated over the sphenoid sinus can be assessed on a sagittal scan.

Usually only a plain CT study is necessary. Contrast enhanced CT scans of the paranasal sinuses are reserved for cases such as tumors and suspected pyoceles. CT cisternography may be used in cases of CSF rhinorrhea. However, a combination of plain CT with T2 weighted MRI images is a better noninvasive option. MRI scans are useful in case of tumors, especially to detect intracranial extension, involvement of soft tissues of the face and to differentiate tumors from secretions. They are also indicated in cases like optic nerve injury and fungal infections of the paranasal sinuses where they give a classical signal void in T2 images. 3-D reconstructed scans help in cases of tumors and craniofacial anomalies. Other radiographic techniques available in our diagnostic armamentarium are the MR angiography, digital subtraction angiography and the dacryocystography. The MR angiography has the advantage of being non-invasive but digital subtraction angiography becomes necessary if any intervention is required in vascular lesions.

Although we can garner a wealth of information from a plain CT paranasal sinus, it sometimes becomes necessary to ask for more advanced investigations to reach a complete diagnosis. Thus, there is an almost bewildering range of technologically advanced investigations available to the endoscopic sinus surgeon. It requires a judicious surgeon to pick and "mix and match" these investigations, in such a way that he gains the maximum information possible at a reasonable cost to the patient.

Anatomical Variations

Exceptions prove the rule...

6 Anatomical Variations

Human beings are individualistic creatures and this is reflected in the human anatomy, which is subject to a large number of anatomical variations or deviations from the rule. The endonasal anatomy is no different and shows numerous variations. These can confound the operating surgeon if he does not have a sound understanding of not only the structure but the genesis of these variations. Certain structures show fairly constant anatomy, e.g. the inferior turbinate and the nasolacrimal duct. Others such as the uncinate process, the frontal recess and the middle turbinate are notorious for their variations.

We will deal with the variations of individual structures in a sequential order.

Septal Deviations

- Septal deviations may occur in an anteroposterior direction in which case they are better appreciated in the axial scans.
- Deviations may also present as sharp spurs at junctions of cartilage with the vomer. These are better seen in coronal scans (Fig. 6.1).

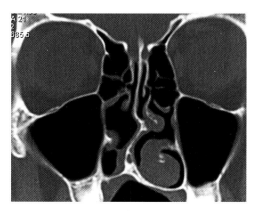

Fig. 6.1: Septal spur

- Septal deviations may compromise key areas like the osteomeatal unit leading to impaired drainage of the sinuses.
- Deviations may also be associated with a concha bullosa or hypertrophied turbinates on the roomy side. These variations in turn may compromise the osteomeatal unit (Fig. 6.2).
- The septum can be pneumatized (Fig. 6.3).

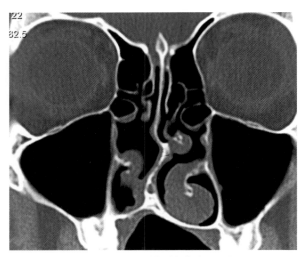

Fig. 6.2: Hypertrophied inferior turbinate

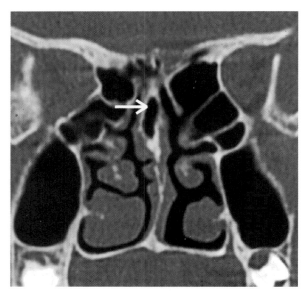

Fig. 6.3: Pneumatization of the septum

Agger Nasi Cell

- The agger nasi cells are usually 1-3 in number. Their size depends on the extent of pneumatization of the lacrimal bone and the adjacent frontonasal process of the maxilla.
- The cells may be hypoplastic.
- They may be very well pneumatized in which case they produce a distinct bulge, anterior to the anterior attachment of the middle turbinate (Fig. 6.4).
- A prominent agger nasi cell tends to displace the anterior attachment of the middle turbinate posterosuperiorly.

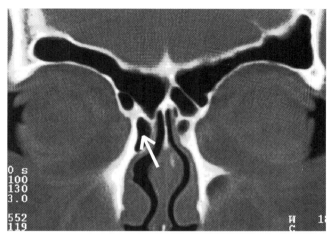

Fig. 6.4: Prominent agger nasi cell

Uncinate Process

- The uncinate process may be hypoplastic or laterally bent. In this case the infundibulum is a narrow space, which may be difficult to enter.
- It may be well developed and medially rotated so much so that it resembles the anterior wall of the bulla. A further medial rotation of the uncinate process brings it in contact with the middle turbinate. Here it may be curled on itself, to look like a duplicated middle turbinate.
- The upper end of the uncinate process may show different patterns of attachment. The commonest type is where the uncinate process attaches laterally to the lamina papyracea; in which case it's upper end encloses within it a blind recess called the recessus terminalis. The commonest mode of drainage of the frontal sinus is medial to the uncinate process (Fig. 6.5A, i and ii).
- The uncinate process may attach to the skull base. In this case the frontal sinus drains into the infundibulum and therefore disease from the frontal sinus can spread to the maxillary sinus and vice versa (Fig. 6.5B, i and ii).
- The uppermost portion of the uncinate process may bend medially to attach to the middle turbinate (Fig. 6.5C, i and ii).
- Occasionally the upper end of the uncinate process may lie free within the middle meatus and not attach to any adjacent bony structure (Fig. 6.5D, i and ii).

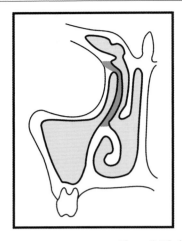 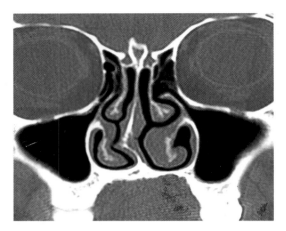

Figs. 6.5A (i) and (ii): Attaching laterally to lamina

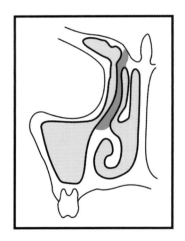 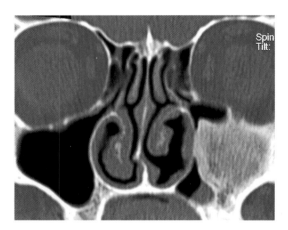

Figs. 6.5B (i) and (ii): Attaching to cribriform plate

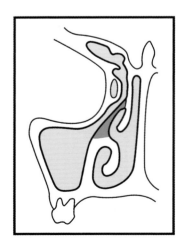 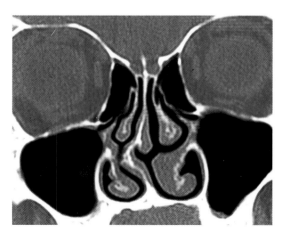

Figs. 6.5C (i) and (ii): Attaching medially to middle turbinate

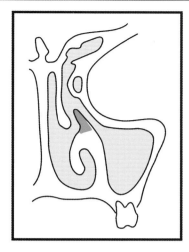 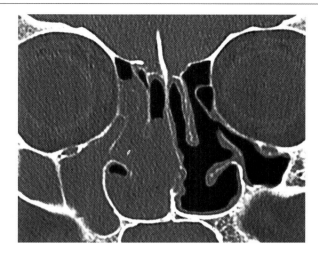

Figs. 6.5D (i) and (ii): Lying free in middle meatus

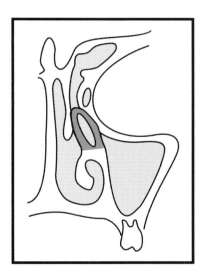 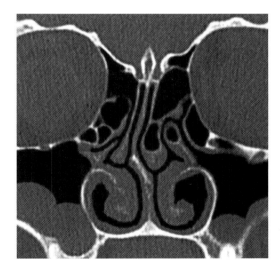

Figs. 6.5E (i) and (ii): Pneumatized uncinate process

- The uppermost portion of the uncinate process may be pneumatized and compromise the infundibulum (Fig. 6.5E, i and ii).
- In pathologic cases the lateral surface of the uncinate facing the infundibulum, will show edematous or polypoidal change indicating infection within the anterior group of sinuses.

Middle Turbinate

- The middle turbinate may be pneumatized and ballooned up. This is a concha bullosa, which is pneumatized from either the frontal recess, the agger nasi cell, anterior ethmoid cells or the middle meatus. The concha bullosa may show isolated disease. It may have septations and therefore multiple cells within it. Although the concha bullosa itself is not considered a pathological finding it may compromise ventilation and drainage of secretions to produce chronic infection of the paranasal sinuses (Fig. 6.6).

- Occasionally the superior meatus may pneumatize the vertical lamella of the middle turbinate to produce what is called the interlamellar cell of Grunwald (Fig. 6.7).
- The middle turbinate may show a sharp bend laterally instead of its usual smooth medial curvature. This is the paradoxically bent middle turbinate. It is quite often bilateral and can block the infundibulum (Fig. 6.8).
- A normally curved middle turbinate may curl upon itself to produce a concavity within it. This concavity is called the turbinate sinus (Fig. 6.9).
- The anterior head of the middle turbinate usually extends upto a few millimeters in front of its anterior attachment to the lateral nasal wall. However, in some cases the anterior head may extend as far anteriorly as 1 cm in front of its anterior attachment. It may be difficult to negotiate the anterior portion of the middle meatus in such a case.

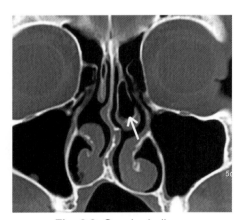

Fig. 6.6: Concha bullosa

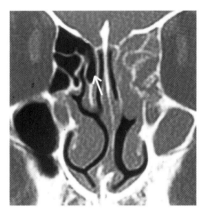

Fig. 6.7: Interlamellar cell

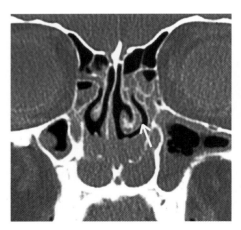

Fig. 6.8: Paradoxically curved middle turbinate

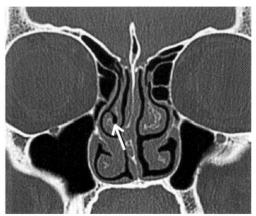

Fig. 6.9: The turbinate sinus

Ethmoidal Bulla

- The ethmoidal bulla is usually the largest and most constantly pneumatized anterior ethmoid cell.
- It may, however, be hypoplastic or rarely even a solid non-pneumatized hillock.
- More commonly it may be extensively pneumatized to produce a large bulge, which abuts against the uncinate process anteriorly or the middle turbinate, compromising the infundibulum or the middle meatus respectively.
- The bulla may not extend upto the skull base, in which case the space between the upper margin of the bulla and the skull base is the suprabullar recess. The suprabullar recess may open into the frontal recess.
- The bulla or its adjacent air cells may not extend upto the ground lamella. This space between the ground lamella and the bulla is called the retrobullar recess.
- Occasionally both the suprabullar and retrobullar recesses are present. They form a semilunar space above and behind the bulla called the sinus lateralis. This sinus lateralis opens into the middle meatus by a cleft, which is called the hiatus semilunaris superioris. The frontal recess may drain into the sinus lateralis.
- The sinus lateralis may extend laterally to pneumatize the roof of the orbit thus forming the supraorbital ethmoid cell. This cell is seen in a coronal CT scan at the level of the bulla behind the frontal sinus (Fig. 6.10).

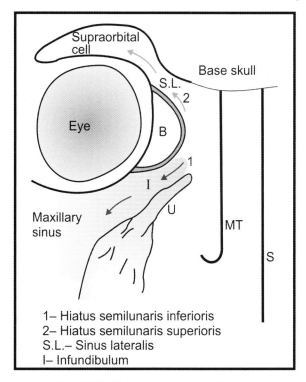

1– Hiatus semilunaris inferioris
2– Hiatus semilunaris superioris
S.L.– Sinus lateralis
I– Infundibulum

Fig. 6.10: Schematic representation at the level of bulla

Ethmoid Air Cells

The anterior and posterior ethmoid air cells may pneumatize surrounding bones like the lacrimal bone, maxilla, frontal bone and sphenoid to produce varying patterns of pneumatization (Figs 6.11A and B). These "migrated" air cells have distinct features and specific names.

- The anterior ethmoid cells pneumatize the lacrimal bone and frontonasal process of the maxilla to produce the agger nasi cells. These cells when well pneumatized produce a distinct bulge on the lateral nasal wall and can compromise the drainage of the frontal recess.
- The anterior ethmoid cells may pneumatize the roof of the maxillary sinus. This migrated cell is the Haller's cell and it is usually seen in the floor of the orbit at the level between the inferior and medial rectus. It can very often compromise the infundibulum (Fig. 6.12).

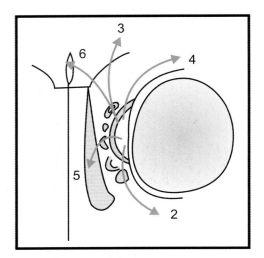 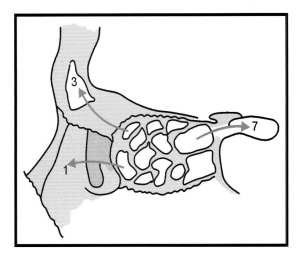

Figs 6.11A and B: Patterns of migration of ethmoidal air cells into: (1) lacrimal bone (agger nasi), (2) inferior to orbit (Haller's cell), (3) frontal bone (frontal cells), (4) supraorbital cell, (5) middle turbinate (concha bullosa), (6) crista galli, (7) above sphenoid (Onodi)

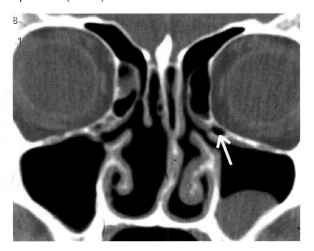

Fig. 6.12: Haller's cell

- The anterior ethmoid cells may migrate into the frontal recess area where they are then named the frontal cells. These are of four types (Figs 6.13A to D):
  — *Type I:* A single cell above the agger nasi cell.
  — *Type II:* Two or more cells above the agger nasi cell.
  — *Type III:* (Frontal bulla) A cell which extends well into the frontal sinus and simulates the frontal sinus itself on endoscopy.
  — *Type IV:* An isolated "loner cell" within the frontal sinus.

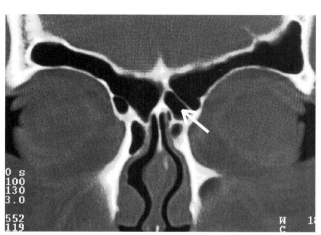

Fig. 6.13A: Frontal cell—type I

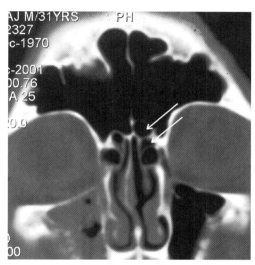

Fig. 6.13B: Frontal cell—type II

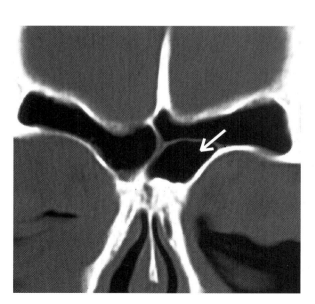

Fig. 6.13C: Frontal cell—type III

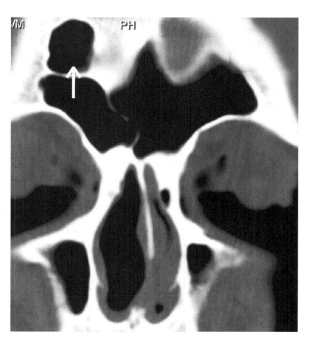

Fig. 6.13D: Frontal cell—type IV

- Pneumatization from the suprabullar recess may extend laterally over the roof of the orbit to form the supraorbital cell. This cell is seen on coronal scans above the ethmoidal bulla and posterior to the frontal sinus (Fig. 6.14).
- Anterior ethmoid cells may pneumatize the middle turbinate to give rise to the concha bullosa.
- Anterior ethmoid cells may also pneumatize the crista galli (Fig. 6.15).
- Posterior ethmoid cells may pneumatize the sphenoid bone posteriorly to give rise to a cell, which extends superolateral to the sphenoid sinus. This is the Onodi cell. The optic nerve and sometimes the internal carotid artery are in close relation with the lateral wall of this cell rather than with the sphenoid sinus (Figs 6.16 and 6.17).

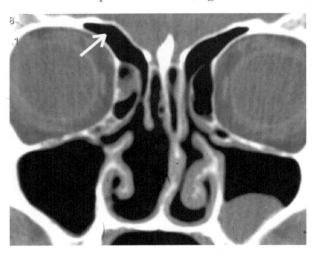

Fig. 6.14: Supraorbital cell

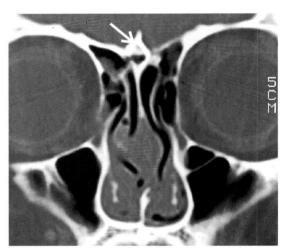

Fig. 6.15: Pneumatization of crista galli

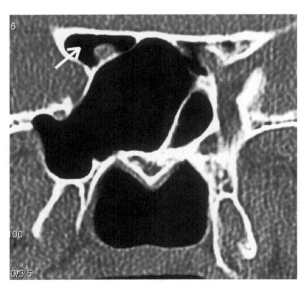

Fig. 6.16: Onodi cell with dehiscent optic nerve

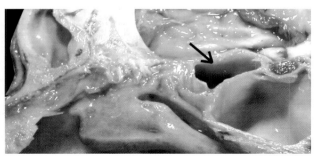

Fig. 6.17: Onodi cell seen in sagittal section

Ground Lamella

- The ground lamella of the middle turbinate, which separates the anterior and posterior ethmoid cells, is not always in a coronal plane. It may bulge into the anterior ethmoids and have a convexity anteriorly. Conversely, it may bulge into the posterior ethmoids with a concavity anteriorly.
- It may show dehiscences or be partially deficient in which case infection can pass from anterior to posterior ethmoids.
- It may itself be pneumatized and split into multiple septae (Fig. 6.18).
- The ground lamella usually attaches to the lamina papyracea. Rarely it may, however, turn inferiorly in which case it *"misses"* the lamina papyracea and attaches to the lateral wall of the maxillary sinus (Fig. 6.19). The maxillary sinus is thus divided into two parts. The posterior part behaves like a posterior ethmoidal cell in terms of drainage and involvement by disease.

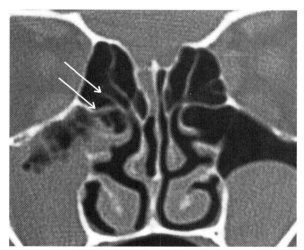

Fig. 6.18: Ground lamella spliting into septae

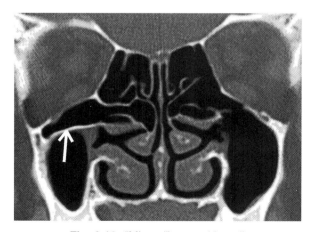

Fig. 6.19: "Missed" ground lamella

Superior/Supreme Turbinate

- The superior turbinate is always present and acts as a guide for the sphenoid ostium.
- It may occasionally be pneumatized (Fig. 6.20) or paradoxically curved (Fig. 6.21).
- A fourth turbinate, i.e. the supreme turbinate, which represents persistence of an ethmoturbinal may be seen in the adult.

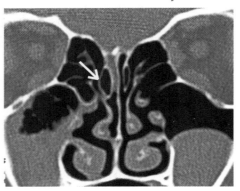 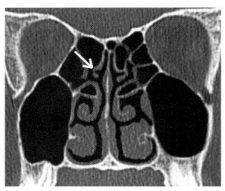

Fig. 6.20: Pneumatized superior turbinate   **Fig. 6.21:** Paradoxically curved superior turbinate

Olfactory Fossa

The olfactory fossa is formed by the horizontal lamella of the cribriform plate, its vertical lamellae and a part of the orbital plate of the frontal bone. The thickness of the orbital plate of the frontal bone is 0.5 mm. The vertical lamella in its thinnest part (where the anterior ethmoidal artery perforates it) is only 1/10th this thickness, i.e. 0.05 mm (Fig. 6.22). The depth of the olfactory fossa varies and has been classified by Keros into (Figs 6.23A, i and ii; B, i and ii; C, i and ii).

- *Type I:* 1-3 mm
- *Type II:* 4-7 mm
- *Type III:* 8-17 mm

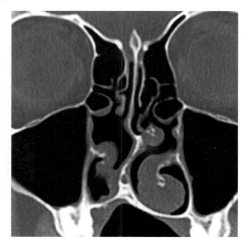

Fig. 6.22: The olfactory fossa

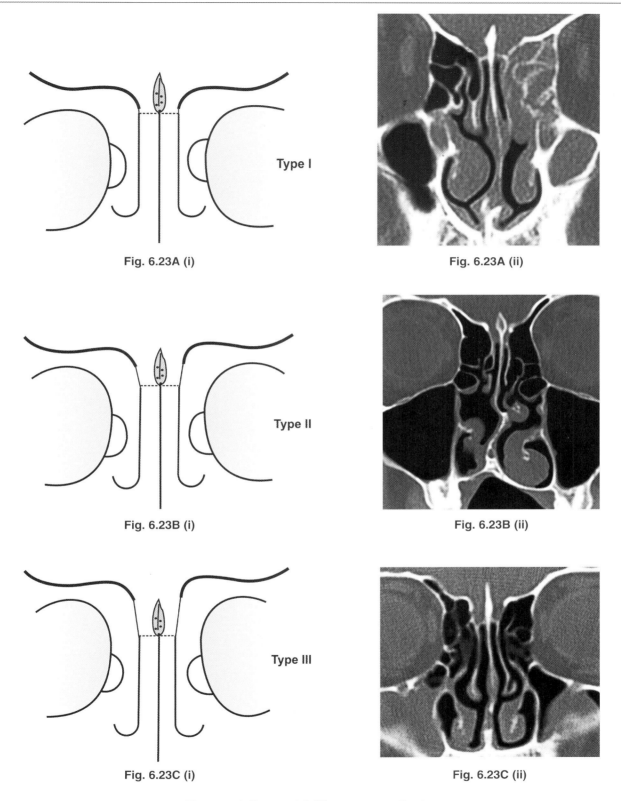

Fig. 6.23A (i)

Fig. 6.23A (ii)

Type I

Fig. 6.23B (i)

Fig. 6.23B (ii)

Type II

Fig. 6.23C (i)

Fig. 6.23C (ii)

Type III

Figs 6.23A (i) to 6.23C (ii): Keros classification

The deeper the olfactory fossa, the longer is the vertical lamella of the cribriform plate. This increased length of very thin bone is liable to injury. However, in a shallow olfactory fossa although the vertical lamella is not very long it is placed in a more horizontal or axial plane and is therefore also liable to injury by the advancing tip of the forceps.

The olfactory fossa is usually symmetrical. Occasionally it may be asymmetrical.

Lamina Papyracea

The orientation of the lamina papyracea is best seen in axial cuts of the CT scan. It runs fairly straight in an anterior to posterior direction between the ethmoid cells and the orbit. It may however, occasionally bend towards the orbit or towards the ethmoid sinus. There may be natural breaks in the lamina papyracea. The edges of these breaks are well corticated as opposed to breaks due to trauma or some expansile lesion.

Sphenoid Sinus

The sphenoid sinus shows great variations in pneumatization (Fig. 6.24).
* It may be present as a small pit in a predominantly non-pneumatized sphenoid bone-conchal type.

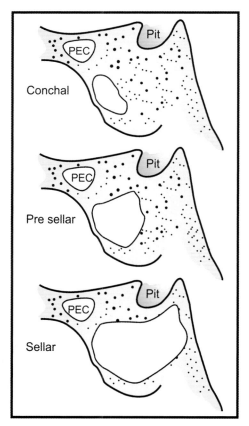

Fig. 6.24: Patterns of sphenoid pneumatization

- It may extend upto the anterior wall of the sella turcica—Presellar type.
- It may pneumatize the entire sphenoid body below and behind the sella turcica, so that the pituitary forms a distinct bulge in its posterosuperior wall—Sellar type.
- Pneumatization may occasionally be different on each side.
- The right and left sphenoid sinuses are more often than not asymmetrical leading to dominance of one sphenoid.
- The intersphenoid septum as well as septae within the sphenoid sinus may attach to vital structures like the optic nerve and the internal carotid artery (Figs 6.25 and 6.26).

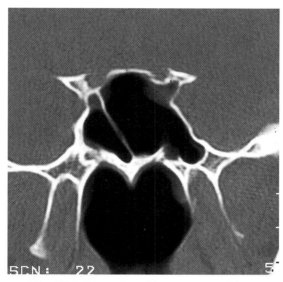

Fig. 6.25: Intersphenoid septum attaching
to optic nerve

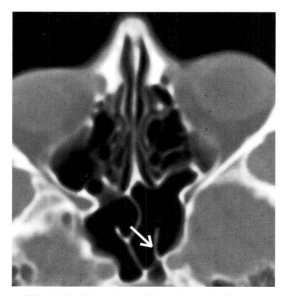

Fig. 6.26: Intersphenoid septum attaching to
internal carotid artery

- Pneumatization of the anterior clinoid process produces a deep recess between the optic nerve and internal carotid artery- the carotico-optic recess. The optic nerve may often be dehiscent in such a case (Fig. 6.27).
- The internal carotid artery may be "clinically dehiscent" (i.e. covered by very thin bone) in 25 percent cases and the optic nerve is dehiscent in about 6 percent cases.
- The sphenoid sinus may show extensive pneumatization laterally into the pterygoid processes and the greater wing of sphenoid. The maxillary and vidian nerves can then be seen prominently within these lateral recesses of the sphenoid (Fig. 6.28).

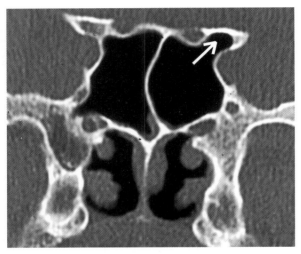

Fig. 6.27: Pneumatized anterior clinoid process

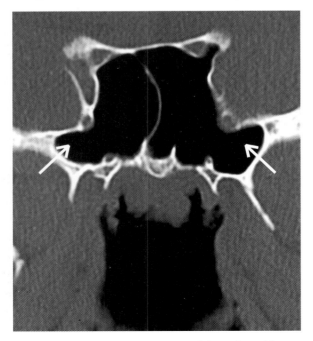

Fig. 6.28: Lateral recesses of the sphenoid

- The sphenoid ostium may be pinpoint, oval or round. It may be easily seen on the anterior face of the sphenoid or may be hidden behind the superior turbinate. Occasionally there may be more than one ostia on one side.
- In a well pneumatized sinus the carotid artery siphon may take a gentle curve or be fairly straight. In elderly individuals the internal carotid artery may take a more tortuous route.

Frontal Sinus

- The frontal sinus may vary from being completely absent to being extensively pneumatized with multiple chambers. These chambers may drain individually into the frontal recess.

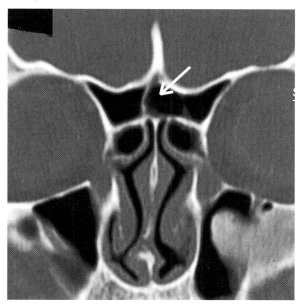

Fig. 6.29: Pneumatized interfrontal septum

- The interfrontal septum may be occasionally pneumatised (Fig. 6.29).
- The pattern of drainage of the frontal sinus as well as different types of frontal cells has already been discussed.

Maxillary Sinus

- The maxillary sinus is fairly constant in its pattern of pneumatization and drainage. Occasionally it may be hypoplastic or asymmetric. Rarely it may be completely absent.
- Partial or complete septations may occur within the maxillary sinus (Fig. 6.30).
- A Haller cell may compromise the infundibulum and the drainage of the maxillary sinus through its normal ostium.
- Accessory ostia may be present in the anterior and posterior fontanelle in 25 percent of the cases.
- An extensively pneumatized maxillary sinus may encroach upon the alveolar process of the maxilla, in which case, the roots of the teeth will

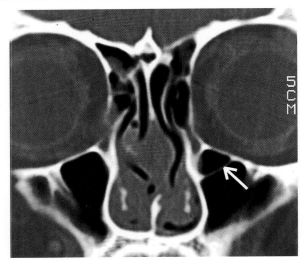

Fig. 6.30: Septa within maxillary sinus

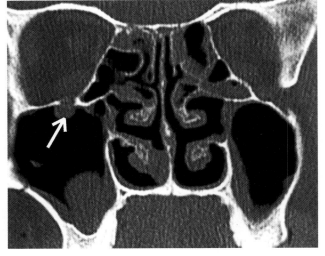

Fig. 6.31: Dehiscent infraorbital nerve

project into the maxillary sinus. Pneumatization may also encroach into the zygomatic process of the maxilla.

- The infraorbital canal may be dehiscent with the nerve lying submucosally (Fig. 6.31).
- The natural ostium is usually ovoid, lies in an oblique plane and appears tunnel like during endoscopy. It may however, be pinpoint, round or multiple.
- The medial wall of the maxillary sinus may be bowed laterally to protrude into the maxillary sinus.

It is now obvious that the nose and paranasal sinuses are subject to many variations in anatomy which are fairly common and not necessarily pathological. As such no surgery is required for these findings on CT scan if the patient is clinically asymptomatic.

They may however be the etiological factor in sinus infections and should be especially looked for when an isolated sinus is involved. For example a type II or III frontal cell may be the only reason for frontal sinusitis and a discerning surgeon would achieve a clinically gratifying result with minimally invasive surgery. More importantly, a sound knowledge of the possible variations would help the surgeon in avoiding pitfalls and harming his patients.

Surgical Anatomy

*"At what point then is the approach of
danger to be expected?"*
Abraham Lincoln (1838)

7 Surgical Anatomy

This chapter is a summary of facts discussed in this book and their relevance in the milieu of the operating theatre.

Diagnostic Endoscopy

- The turbinates and septum are very sensitive to touch; it is therefore necessary to get good decongestion and anesthesia of the nose prior to attempting diagnostic endoscopy.
- Endoscopy should be done in such a way so as to avoid touching the septum and turbinates during the passes. The second pass can prove to be the most difficult as the sphenoethmoidal recess is a narrow niche.

The Septum

- In case of a deviated nasal septum or a nasal spur, diagnostic endoscopy should be done in the roomy nostril first so as to gain the patient's confidence prior to attempting endoscopy in the narrow cavity.
- A very common site for mucosal trauma and subsequent adhesions is on the opposing surfaces of a septal spur and the inferior turbinate. Special care should be exercised to prevent trauma to these opposing mucosal surfaces.

Olfactory Fossa

- The olfactory fossa is most often symmetrical bilaterally. In case of a break in the horizontal portion of the cribriform plate, the meninges may descend into the upper recesses of the nasal cavity. The olfactory fossa will appear asymmetrical on coronal CT scans. This is called the *gyrus rectus sign* and is indicative of the site of breach in a case of CSF rhinorrhea.
- The olfactory nerves pass through the cribriform plate to reach the nasal cavity. These foramina may appear like breaks in the detailed 1 mm coronal

CT scans, which may be taken to locate a site of CSF leak. This fact should be borne in mind when hunting for a CSF leak.

Lacrimal Apparatus

- The lateral wall of the nasolacrimal duct is formed by the frontonasal process of the maxilla which is thick bone. The medial wall however is formed by thin bones, namely, the descending portion of the lacrimal bone and the lacrimal process of the inferior turbinate. Thus contrary to common belief, the nasolacrimal duct can be injured without encountering thick bone whilst widening the maxillary ostium anteriorly.
- The lacrimal bone articulates superiorly with the frontal bone which is very thick. Therefore, in exposing the upper portion of the lacrimal sac one may need to use a drill on this bone.
- The lacrimal fossa does not extend backwards beyond the lacrimal bone. Hence in endoscopic dacryocystorhinostomy one needs to operate anterior to the uncinate process and it is therefore not necessary to remove the uncinate process.
- Since canalization of the nasolacrimal duct is not complete till after birth, regurgitation of tears is common in infancy. This problem does not need to be addressed surgically in most cases.
- A rare anomaly of the lacrimal system is the oblique facial cleft in which the maxillary process does not fuse with the lateral nasal process and the nasolacrimal duct is not formed.

Uncinate Process

- The upper part of the uncinate process is hidden by the attachment of the middle turbinate. Therefore an uncinectomy by any technique does not remove this uppermost portion. It needs to be removed separately with a ballpoint probe or forceps while dissecting in the region of the frontal recess.
- In a hypoplastic and laterally rotated uncinate process the infundibulum is very shallow. If uncinectomy is done with a sickle knife in such a case it is easy to traverse the infundibulum and enter the orbit accidentally.
- It is not necessary to remove the entire uncinate process in all cases. For example only the horizontal portion of the uncinate process needs to be removed if there is isolated disease of the maxillary sinus.

Middle Turbinate

- At least two of the three attachments of the middle turbinate (namely, the anterior and the posterior attachment) should be preserved to maintain its stability. Preservation of the lower border of the ground lamella also helps to keep the middle turbinate stable and prevents its lateralization.
- The middle turbinate should be manipulated very gently as it attaches directly to the cribriform plate. A forcible attempt to medialize the middle turbinate in order to get a better view of the middle meatus may lead to a break in the cribriform plate and a CSF leak.

- While dissecting in the region of the frontal recess, care should be taken to maintain the mucosa over the middle turbinate. If the mucosa of the anterior attachment of the middle turbinate is stripped off, adhesions will form between the lateral nasal wall and the upper attachment of the middle turbinate. These adhesions will cause lateralization of the middle turbinate and obliteration of the frontal recess with subsequent iatrogenic frontal sinus disease. In extreme cases complete obliteration of the middle meatus may occur.
- Preserving the posterior attachment of the middle turbinate to the perpendicular plate of the ethmoid protects the sphenopalatine artery as it exits from the sphenopalatine foramen just above and behind the posterior attachment of the middle turbinate.
- While opening a concha bullosa care should be taken to maintain the mucosa over its lateral surface, so as to prevent adhesions developing between the two opposing raw areas.

Bulla Ethmoidalis

- Clearance of the bulla, anterior and posterior ethmoid cells should be done using the side of the straight or upward biting forceps and not the tip in order to prevent accidental injury to the lamina papyracea and orbital contents.
- The anterior wall of the bulla lies just in front of the anterior ethmoidal artery at the base skull. Thus, if the bulla is kept intact during dissection in the frontal recess area, the risk of bleeding from the anterior ethmoidal artery is minimized.
- Minimal inflammation in the osteomeatal area can block off aeration to the anterior ethmoid, frontal and the maxillary sinus, leading to infection in them. This concept is the basis of Messerklinger's functional endoscopic sinus surgery whereby the clearance of this area alone may reverse changes in the draining sinuses.

Maxillary Ostium

- The normal maxillary sinus ostium lies deep in the infundibulum very close to the attachment of the uncinate process to the lateral wall. If the entire width of the uncinate process is not removed the normal ostium can be missed during dissection. This leads to the "missed ostium sequence" and recirculation of mucus.
- The presence of accessory ostia also leads to recirculation of mucus. The mucus is transported out of the sinus through the normal ostia and reenters the sinus through an accessory ostium. This recirculation of mucus can be prevented by joining the normal ostium with the accessory ostium so as to get one large opening.
- The normal ostium should be widened in an anteroinferior direction at the expense of the anterior fontanelle to prevent injury to the nasolacrimal duct, which lies 5 mm anterior to it.
- The lamina papyracea and the orbit lie just above the maxillary ostium. Hence, if for some reason the normal ostium cannot be located, it is safest to probe for the maxillary sinus ostium just above the inferior turbinate.

The probe should be directed in an anteroinferior direction. This would prevent accidental entry into the orbit.

- A branch of the sphenopalatine artery runs along the lateral nasal wall in the middle meatus. This branch may be encountered whilst widening the maxillary ostium posteriorly.

Frontal Recess

- The path of drainage of the frontal sinus depends upon the mode of attachment of the uncinate process. If the uncinate process is attached to the cribriform plate the frontal sinus will drain into the infundibulum. If the uncinate process is attached to the lamina papyracea, the frontal sinus drains medial to the infundibulum. In such a case the infundibulum will lead up into a blind recess—the recessus terminalis. The dome of this recess has to be removed before the frontal sinus can be entered. This has been described by Stammberger as 'uncapping the egg'. Care should be taken to direct the probe laterally as the thin vertical lamella of the cribriform plate lies medially.

- Whilst dissecting in the frontal recess the surgeon may think he has entered the frontal sinus, when in fact, he is within a frontal cell. It is necessary to de-roof this frontal cell so as to reach the frontal sinus and establish its drainage.

- When a supraorbital cell is present the frontal recess will show two openings. In this case, the medial one is the frontal sinus opening and the lateral one is the opening of the supraorbital cell.

- When the frontal sinus drains medial to the uncinate process, its secretions do not traverse the infundibulum. Thus infection from the frontal sinus would not normally spread to the maxillary sinus and vice versa. However, if the frontal sinus drains lateral to the uncinate process its secretions pass through the infundibulum making the maxillary sinus prone to infection.

- When the frontal recess is viewed from below with an endoscope, the opening of the frontal sinus can be seen in the anterior limits of the frontal recess. We have to look around the corner of the frontal beak in order to view the interior of the frontal sinus. This is best done with a 70° or 45° telescope or by hyper extending the head whilst using a 0° telescope.

Ethmoidal Air Cells

- The anterior ethmoidal air cells are variable in number; the posterior ethmoidal air cells are fewer and larger. The ground lamella should be perforated slightly medially and inferiorly in order to enter the posterior ethmoid air cells. This will prevent accidental entry into the orbit.

- As the surgeon dissects posteriorly, he must learn to recognize the posterior most pyramidal ethmoidal cell. He must then change the direction of surgery inferomedially to access the sphenoid sinus. If he continues to dissect through the posterior wall of the posterior ethmoid he would enter the cranial cavity.

Lamina Papyracea

A breach in the lamina papyracea anteriorly may not cause major damage because a pad of fat separates the medial rectus from the lamina papyracea. Posteriorly, however, the medial rectus is in close relation to the lamina papyracea and therefore is more prone to injury.

After the lamina papyracea is cleared of cells and the maxillary ostium is widened a "ridge" can be delineated and extrapolated backwards. This ridge can be used as a landmark to open the sphenoid sinus.

Sphenoid Sinus

- Differentiation between the posterior most ethmoid cell and the sphenoid sinus is one of the most common difficulties faced by the novice endoscopic surgeon. The following points help to identify the sphenoid sinus:
  — The sphenoid sinus is globular in shape (like the inside of a pot). The posterior most ethmoid cell on the other hand is pyramidal in shape and tapers to an apex posteriorly.
  — The sphenoid sinus opens inferior to the maxillary ridge mentioned above in a more or less axial plane. The posterior ethmoid cells most often open above the ridge in a coronal plane.
  — The roof of the posterior choana and the posterior end of the septum can be used as landmarks to identify the normal sphenoid ostium and then widen it to open the sinus.
- The sphenoid ostium lies close to the roof of the sphenoid sinus. Therefore it is safest to widen the ostium in an inferior direction along its anterior wall. A branch of the sphenopalatine artery runs across the anterior face of the sphenoid to reach the septum. This may be injured during widening the ostium. This bleeding is safely and effectively controlled using a monopolar suction cautery. Another technique is to raise a mucosal flap along with the artery and nibble away only the bone of the anterior wall so as to prevent damage to the artery.
- Since the skull base slopes downward from anterior to posterior, its lowest level is the roof of the sphenoid. This fact should be borne in mind while clearing the cells of the ethmoid fovea.
- There is a great deal of unnecessary nervousness on the part of the beginner, in approaching the sphenoid sinus laterally through the posterior ethmoid cells. If a curved ballpoint or suction is used to probe inferomedially through the posterior ethmoid cell, this instrument can go only in one of two areas, i.e. either the sphenoid sinus or more anteriorly into the nasal cavity. A common mistake by the beginner is to probe more anteriorly and therefore reenter the nasal cavity itself instead of the sphenoid sinus. This can be easily rectified by probing in an inferior direction in a more posterior cell. Thus if the direction of dissection is strictly inferomedially it is not possible for the surgeon to damage any vital structure or to accidentally enter the cranial cavity. The risk for these mishaps exists only if the surgeon dissects in a posterior, superior or lateral direction.
- In approximately 6 percent of cases, the bone over the optic nerve may be dehiscent and in approximately 25 percent of cases, bone over the internal

carotid artery may be clinically dehiscent. This may be difficult to visualize on CT scan, if the sphenoid sinus is full of polyps. Therefore extreme caution has to be exercised in pulling polyps out from within the sphenoid sinus.

Anterior and Posterior Ethmoidal Arteries

- The orbitocranial canal may have bony dehiscences (40%), which leave the anterior ethmoidal artery exposed to the risk of trauma.
- The point at which the anterior ethmoidal artery perforates the lateral lamella of the cribriform plate is the thinnest part of the anterior base skull (0.05 mm). The underlying dura is also strongly adherent to this area of bone. Thus this region is particularly vulnerable to iatrogenic CSF leaks. Patients with deep olfactory fossae with long lateral lamellae (Keros type III) are at the greatest risk. However, as mentioned earlier, shallow olfactory fossae can also be vulnerable to injury as the lateral lamella is more horizontal in orientation, and therefore, more easily accessible to the tip of the advancing forceps.
- Viewed from the side of the orbit, the anterior and posterior ethmoidal arteries enter the nose at the level of the suture line between the frontal bone and the lamina papyracea. The distance from the anterior lacrimal crest to the anterior ethmoidal artery is 24 mm (anterior ethmoidal foramen), from the anterior ethmoidal artery to the posterior ethmoidal artery is 12 mm (posterior ethmoidal foramen) and from the posterior ethmoidal artery to the optic nerve is 6 mm (optic foramen).

Sphenopalatine Artery

The sphenopalatine artery can be approached through the posterior part of the middle meatus by detaching the middle turbinate from the ethmoidal crest so as to access the sphenopalatine foramen.

In Conclusion...

This is really for my junior colleagues and for all those who are starting out in endoscopic surgery – testing the waters, so to speak.

One often hears of the *learning curve* in endoscopic sinus surgery. I think of the 4 lamellae the surgeon has to cross during surgery, as the 4 stages in his learning curve. He first learns to do diagnostic endoscopies and possibly just an uncinectomy. Having developed hand-eye coordination and some knowledge of the anatomy, he would then breach the anterior wall of the bulla to operate on the anterior group of sinuses. Once he has gained enough experience, only then should he breach the ground lamella to operate on the posterior group of sinuses. This is because the complications arising from surgery on the posterior group of sinuses are far more debilitating as compared to those in the anterior group of sinuses.

Having mastered surgery in the posterior group of sinuses, the surgeon would then venture beyond the sinus boundaries to the orbit, the cranial cavity and the pterygopalatine fossa.

We all trace our own learning curve. The important thing is to recognize that it exists and that to ignore it or to jump it would be to court disaster. However, if we combine a sound knowledge of the subject with meticulousness and patience the results will definitely be gratifying for our patients.

Index

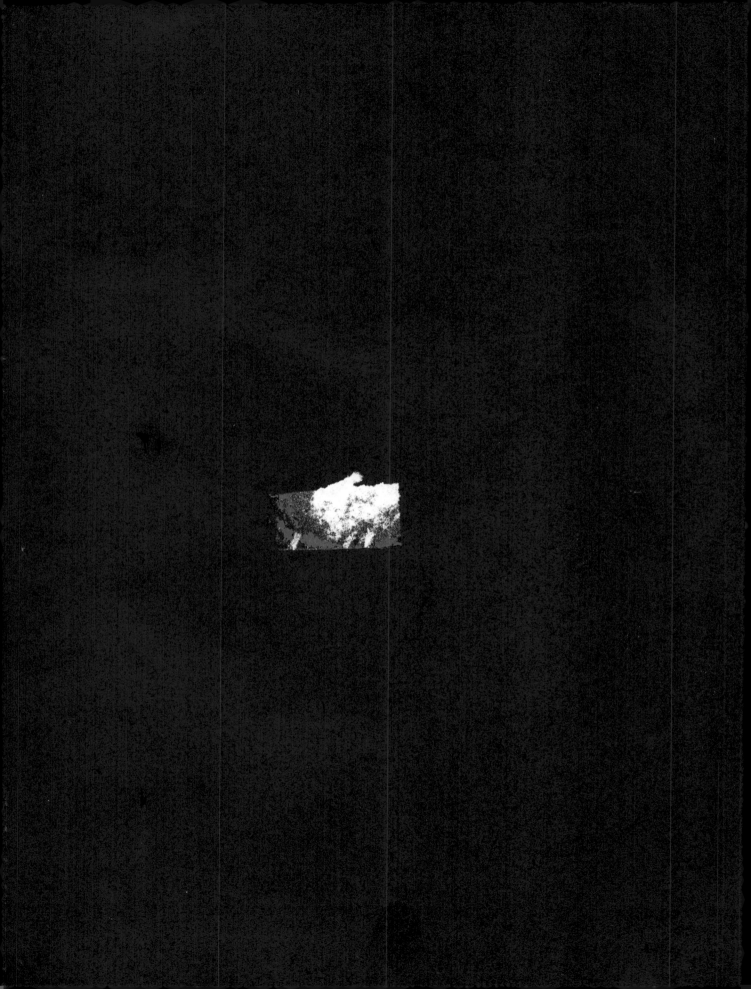